Yogic Tools for Recovery Workbook

YOGIC TOOLS
for Recovery
WORKBOOK

KYCZY HAWK

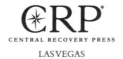

CRP
CENTRAL RECOVERY PRESS
LAS VEGAS

Central Recovery Press (CRP) is committed to publishing exceptional materials addressing addiction treatment, recovery, and behavioral healthcare topics.

For more information, visit www.centralrecoverypress.com.

Publisher: Central Recovery Press
            3321 N. Buffalo Drive
            Las Vegas, NV 89129

23 22 21 20 19 18   1 2 3 4 5

ISBN: 978-1-942094-63-0 (print)
       978-1-942094-64-7 (e-book)

Photo of Kyczy Hawk by William Hawk. Used with permission.

The Twelve Steps of Narcotics Anonymous. Reprinted by permission of NA World Services, Inc. All rights reserved. The Twelve Steps of NA reprinted for adaptation by permission of A.A. World Services, Inc.

Translation of Sutra 1.14, 2.28, 2.33, 2.35, 2.36, and 2.44: *The Yoga Sutras of Patanjali* by Gary Kissiah. Copyright Lilalabs Publishing LLC, 2016.

Translation of Sutra 1.32: Used with permission from Reverend Jaganath Carrera.

Translation of Sutra 1.2 and 3.36: *Miracle in Progress: A Handbook for Holistic Recovery* by Marta Mrotek, 2014.

Translation of Sutra 2.28 and 4.30: Kyczy Hawk.

Page 29: "Poem XXVI" from *Songs of Kabir* translated by Rabindranath Tagore, 1915. Public domain.

Pages 74 and 79: *The Yoga Sutras of Patanjali* by Gary Kissiah. Copyright Lilalabs Publishing LLC, 2016.

Every attempt has been made to contact copyright holders. If copyright holders have not been properly acknowledged, please contact us. Central Recovery Press will be happy to rectify the omission in future printings of this book.

Publisher's Note: This book contains general information about yoga, addiction, addiction recovery, and related matters. The information is not medical advice. This book is not an alternative to medical advice from your doctor or other professional healthcare provider. Our books represent the experiences and opinions of their authors only. Every effort has been made to ensure that events, institutions, and statistics presented in our books as facts are accurate and up-to-date. To protect their privacy, the names of some of the people, places, and institutions in this book may have been changed.

Cover and interior design and layout by Sara Streifel, Think Creative Design

TABLE OF CONTENTS

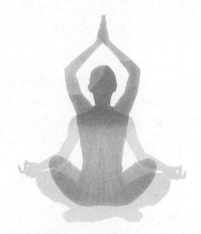

INTRODUCTION

It matters not which one of the twelve-step programs you call home. Your journey may have brought you to more than one program after having discovered that addiction has affected you in more that one way. You may also be in a relationship with one or more people who are afflicted with this disease.

In its most obvious mode, addiction is substance abuse—tobacco, alcohol, or other drugs—but this disease comes in many forms and manifests in behaviors, such as gambling, sexual activity, shopping, and debt, or loving addicts and having become impaired through that love. All forms of addiction have multiple impacts, and the Twelve Steps can help you discover what these impacts are.

Addiction is a disease of separation. It will separate you from your money, friends, family, job, home, dignity, and soul. If addiction goes unchecked, it will separate you from your life. However, using yoga practices can assist you as you reunify yourself inside and out.

How to Use This Workbook

Welcome to the action portion of *Yogic Tools for Recovery*. In this workbook, you will record your yoga and recovery process, which is a concrete way to work the steps. As a companion to the book *Yogic Tools for Recovery: A Guide for Working the Twelve Steps,* this workbook is not intended as a stand-alone guide, although it could be used as such. My other books, *Yoga and the Twelve-Step Path* and *Yogic Tools for Recovery,* provide a deeper investigation into yogic concepts and philosophies.

Each section of this workbook focuses on one of the Twelve Steps and guides you using yoga concepts as you prepare for the step and work it. The practices follow the feelings and impressions inside you as you discover how your addiction, or your adaptation to the addiction of someone else, has become part of you. The investigation can then show you how you can embody your new recovery-oriented self.

Take your time with each step; this isn't a race. Keep in mind there are no right or wrong answers and not all sections will apply to all people. Challenge yourself to write more than a yes or no answer to the sections that do apply. Noting examples and details will enrich your experience. It may also help you recall those specific circumstances more vividly if and when you refer back to a step as you complete a subsequent one.

Each of you is being called upon by your universal spirit, or higher power, to redo the steps in this manner at a various point in your recovery. Where you are emotionally, spiritually, and in your life circumstances will have an impact on how this process flows for you. Avoid comparing yourself and your journey to others. Find contentment in your own path.

This yogic journey shouldn't be your first time through the steps. *Yogic Tools for Recovery* and this companion workbook are designed for someone working the steps again, after first having taken them in the prescribed fashion of his or her primary fellowship. If this is your first exposure to the Twelve Steps, it could cause you some confusion with your primary program. I recommend using this workbook at a later time when you are going through the steps for an additional time, focusing on your primary addiction or working with an underlying issue or newly arising addiction.

Having completed the steps as a member of the Al-Anon fellowship, I can attest to their efficacy. If you are the child of an addict, in relationship with someone in active addiction, or with someone in recovery, you will find the steps useful. The brain of a coaddict, the loved one of an addict, changes in the same ways the brain of an addict changes. The nervous system goes through similar adaptations to constant stress. The way out of the damage and the road to wholeness is also the same. Doing the steps with the yogic perspective will encourage you, too, to become more familiar with yourself and heal in a deeper way.

The language in this book is directed primarily to the addict and for simplicity has been left that way. Each of the topics and questions can be gently "translated" into phrases that apply to having a relationship with an addict: the emotions and behaviors that we adopt in order to manage our environment and our feelings. There is a substantial loss of self resulting from being in a relationship with someone who uses or has used or had destructive behaviors or who is recovering from them. When there is a phrase that begins, for example, "How has your addiction…," you can amend that to read "How has your relationship with an addict…." Read the content and the questions loosely and repurpose them to be meaningful to you and your situation.

Many of us in recovery have discovered that we are "double winners" meaning that we are members of both rooms, the room/program of the recovering addict and the room/program of those who are in relationship with addicts. I am. I discovered that being a child of an alcoholic was the primary form of the disease that I needed to address for my full recovery. If you find this is true for you, you may complete this workbook from that perspective as well.

Be certain that you keep that single addiction—process or behavior—in mind as you do the steps. As you go through the steps, keep your focus on whatever manifestation you want to address. It can be easy to stray from one vexing behavior to another as you go from step to step. See how steady you can be in following your initial intention, or add the new process to Step One and go from there. The steps can then be repeated to address another behavior or issue. For example, a person may start doing the steps focusing on his codependency issues, particularly as they relate to his job or career. Halfway through the steps, he starts focusing on negative self-talk and self-limiting beliefs. At this point, he has veered off the issue of codependency and onto his own habits of negative thinking. First, he should do the steps focusing on his job situation. Then, he should do them again focusing on his unhealthy thinking behaviors.

Just as there is a pose for everyone—a yoga pose that feels right using the proper balance of effort and ease—there may be a part of working the steps that feels more comfortable. For example, when you find yourself in a yoga pose, one that isn't enjoyable, it feels like work and discomfort. This is similar to feeling some attraction to one step and a certain resistance to another. Noting this resistance or affinity is also an important part of the journey and is a necessary part of the recovery process.

If there is something you are not ready to investigate, you can pause, make a note in the margin of this workbook, proceed, and come back to it. Rather than assuming that something doesn't apply at all, make a commitment to return to that portion and check it out after some days have passed. You may be surprised. Or, you may find that you really have nothing to expand upon in that area. This, too, is an important piece of information for your journey.

Meditations appear throughout this workbook, and you can read them by yourself or read them aloud if you are working with another person or in a group. Some of the meditations are available online at www.centralrecoverypress.com.

Charts and explanations of the main yoga terms are available in the Appendix. These are my interpretations and are not the only definitions. I have combined my research, training, and work with others and compiled explanations that I have found useful when working the steps and expanding my recovery. Yoga has broad applications and usefulness, so there is much more to be divined from the philosophy than what I have presented here. Please enjoy your own research and investigations. Your inquiry will personalize and augment its usefulness to you.

When I designed this material, I disciplined myself to do each step in sequence as it is suggested. It was surprising what came up for me. I had glossed over some connections, sensations, and commitments. I also noticed where I truly retained control of the outcome and where I avoided reaching out to my universal spirit. This was my experience, and you will have your own; however, try to let go of expectations or a specific outcome, just a little, and approach this work with a beginner's mind.

Be kind to yourself as you move through this process. You are doing something familiar in an unfamiliar way. Some parts may feel natural; others may feel contrived. Let go of the "contempt prior to investigation," a phrase coined by philosopher Hebert Spencer, that may block you.

I wish you well as you welcome your true self home and blessings as you embark on this yogic journey.

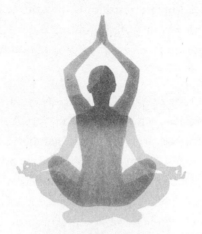

STEP ONE

We admitted that we were powerless over our addiction,
that our lives had become unmanageable.

RECOVERY CONCEPTS

Honesty, Acceptance, Surrender

GUIDING YOGIC PRINCIPLE

"When the yogini is firmly established in truthfulness,
she attains the fruits of actions without acting."

SUTRA 2.36

Before you begin Step One, please pause and take a few slow, deep breaths. This is an example of centering, grounding, and breathing, a tool that will come in handy throughout this workbook and in life in general. After you complete reading to the end of this paragraph, close your eyes; take three, long, slow breaths; notice your seated position, the sounds around you, and your mind chatter—without criticism or adjustment—and then take an additional three breaths. When done, open your eyes and resume your work.

Recall what you read in Chapter One of *Yogic Tools for Recovery: A Guide for Working the Twelve Steps*. Most likely this is not your first time going through the steps. You may be dealing with an issue that was uncovered when you stopped drinking, using, gambling, smoking, or any other form of addiction that drew you to this work. Or, you may have become aware of something that is causing you discomfort, something that is compelling you to make erroneous and painful decisions over and over. It could also be a new obsession or compulsion addiction coming to the surface, such as disordered eating, spending, or codependency-infused relationships.

Before you begin working the steps, please answer the following questions. Your responses can take any written form. If you need more room to write, you may find using a journal beneficial.

What is causing trouble in your life?

What is having a negative impact on your family, friends, work, relationships, health, purpose, and journey in life?

What craving or desire is blocking you from your spiritual self?

To be certain that you remain centered on the purpose for doing the steps at this time, it is important to remain focused on what brings you to do this work. What is the topic you are investigating while doing the steps this time?

Considering the term *powerless,* please note how you have tried, stumbled, and then failed to exert power over this process or issue. Recall some attempts in detail and write them down.

You will start by using the *yamas,* or the restraints, as you examine powerlessness and its companion: the need to control. Consider the ethic of *ahimsa*, or non-harming.

How has non-harming been *disregarded* as you struggle with powerlessness?

When struggling with the illusion of managing your life while in active addiction, how have you harmed yourself?

Today, when struggling with the illusion of managing your life while acting on an obsession and/or compulsion, how are you harming yourself?

How have you harmed others?

What about *satya*, or non-lying? Has lying been a part of your struggle with powerlessness or unmanageability?

Addiction—whether it is a behavior, such as rage, lust, or spending, or a substance, such as drugs, alcohol, or sugar—is by nature a violation of the ethics of *brahmacharya,* or non-excess, and *aparigraha,* or non-attachment.

Specifically, how have the qualities of powerlessness and/or unmanageability impacted the principles of non-excess and non-attachment?

Next, you will investigate your identified issue using the *koshas*—the five layers of our being—as well as the *kleshas*—the five sources of mental torment or sufferings—to examine your experience of powerlessness. Take a few moments, closing your eyes, and remember what it has been like trying to control your addiction. Perhaps, remember times you have bargained with yourself in order to control or quit, saying things, such as "Just one more time"; "I will only use (or stop using) if this happens or that doesn't happen"; "If someone does or doesn't do something"; or "If I live here or have that job."

> Bring your attention inward and remember how your body felt at these times when you were bargaining and when you broke this agreement. Was there tightness or contraction? Did you feel something in your back, neck, or jaw? Did you feel a sensation in other parts of your body? You may recall sensations or you may not. You may not have had feelings. You may just feel numb. Explain how you felt.

Whether your addiction is to people, substances, or behaviors, you experience the phenomenon of craving, the desire to engage in something in a degree that is beyond all reason. You may feel compelled to please others and be involved in their lives to the detriment of your own. You may spend your last dollar and your future dollars on things, hands of cards, or drugs and risk financial ruin. You may expose your family and those you love to the risk of financial ruin by using, gambling, or starving yourself to a life-threatening extent. You do this when you don't want to; you do this when you know it is incorrect and dangerous. You do this when you promise not to. This is how you know you are powerless.

> Thinking that you have control is erroneous thinking, and this is the root of your suffering called *avidya,* or false understanding. What were some of the illusions you have held regarding your addiction?

Describe your experiences with craving, also known as *raga*.

How does/did craving affect your koshas?

- Your physical layer

- Your energy layer

- Your mental/emotional layer

- Your wisdom layer or your character

- Your spiritual bliss layer

Think about how *dvesha,* or aversion or avoidance, has impacted your choices in regards to being powerless over your addiction. Perhaps, you avoided social discomfort or awkwardness, or the pain of past events felt overwhelming. Maybe you didn't want to feel abandoned, so you manifested codependent behaviors. Withdrawal may cause worry or concern and may even have physical repercussions, which can also be something you want to avoid.

Has the aversion of the unpleasant emotional discomfort and/or anticipated pain of withdrawal caused you to continue some behavior or substance? Withdrawal applies to alcohol and other drugs, sugar, and other substances as well as many behaviors, such as compulsive use of sex or unhealthy relationships.

How does/did aversion or avoidance affect your koshas?

- Your physical layer

- Your energy layer

- Your mental/emotional layer

- Your wisdom layer or your character

- Your spiritual layer

In recovery, we often experience a fear of death, change, or transformation, also known as *abhinivesha*. (The devil we know is often preferred to the one we don't.) We step into the unknown and perhaps begin to fear losing that which we know, are familiar with, and at some level understand. Change can feel overwhelming, and this discomfort occurs over and over as we peel the onion layers of ourselves and delve deeper into the sources of our suffering.

How has your fear of change impacted your understanding of powerlessness?

How does/did your fear of change affect your koshas?

- Your physical layer

- Your energy layer

- Your mental/emotional layer

- Your wisdom layer or your character

- Your spiritual bliss layer

As you consider powerlessness, your *asmita,* or false ego, will step in your way. We each have our persona, our roles in life, the way we think others see us, and the way we want to present ourselves to others. We may identify with a single aspect of ourselves and fear that if this were to go away there would be nothing left of us.

These ideas are based on a story, or many stories, that we have about ourselves. These stories have some truth, but also they are based on a false understanding (*avidya*) of who we are. This is particularly true when it comes to addiction.

> How has your ego—your unclear and perhaps untrue sense of self—influenced your ability to admit powerlessness in regards to your addiction?

How does/did false ego affect your koshas?

- Your physical layer

- Your energy layer

- Your mental/emotional layer

- Your wisdom layer or your character

- Your spiritual layer

In this next section, you are going to consider the *chakras*. Our energy centers record our impressions and our feelings. We are also influenced by the qualities of our energy centers. Unmanageability will have caused some chakras to be out of balance. Out of balance chakras will have had a negative influence on how you handle events in your life. They are interrelated. You will dig deeper into the chakras at each step, so for now focus on how they relate to powerlessness and unmanageability.

How has active addiction/compulsion impacted the energy flow in the following chakras? (Refer to the How Chakras Affect Your Body in the Appendix to help you answer this question.)

ROOT CHAKRA

- Overactive

- Underactive

SACRAL CHAKRA

- Overactive

- Underactive

SOLAR PLEXUS CHAKRA

- Overactive

- Underactive

HEART CHAKRA

- Overactive

- Underactive

THROAT CHAKRA

- Overactive

- Underactive

THIRD EYE CHAKRA
- Overactive

- Underactive

CROWN CHAKRA
- Overactive

- Underactive

The First Step sets the stage for future work and healing. In traditional yoga therapy, this is known as "defining the problem." We can't move forward effectively until we evaluate where we are. These exercises, using the lens of yoga to look at the First Step, will assist you in setting the focus for your study.

Over time, your comprehension of the yoga concepts will become more fluid. The language will become easier, and the underlying tenets will become more understandable as you move forward, one step at a time.

After doing this internal review and introspection, take ten minutes to get grounded once again. You can do this by doing a legs up the wall pose or taking a walk outside in the fresh air.

POSE

If you choose to do the Your Legs Up the Wall pose, you can refer to the process in Chapter One of *Yogic Tools for Recovery* or follow the guidance provided in a short video at www.centralrecoverypress.com.

MEDITATION

If you choose to take a walk, consider a walking meditation where you take the time to feel each footstep. Use your senses as you look around and listen to the ambient sounds where you are. If you are hiking, determine if you can discern the smells of plants, flowers, leaves, or soil. Experience the air and temperature on your skin. Be alive and part of the universe—a walking meditation.

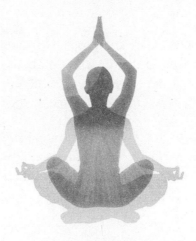

STEP TWO

We came to believe that a Power
greater than ourselves could restore us to sanity.

RECOVERY CONCEPTS

Hope, Faith

GUIDING YOGIC PRINCIPLE

"Yoga is the stilling or the quieting of the fluctuations,
the misinterpretations of the mind."

SUTRA 1.2

After reading Chapter Two in *Yogic Tools for Recovery: A Guide for Working the Twelve Steps,* you can move on to finding or reconnecting with a higher power and opening you heart to the possibility of care.

At this point in recovery, you hopefully have come to understand and accept that you have become unhealthy, unwhole, or even unbalanced due to, and in relation to, your addiction. The solution can't come from within the mind at its current state. Consider the words of Albert Einstein: "We cannot solve our problems with the same thinking we used when we created them."

The solution can't come without some form of intervention such as the wise words of others—good orderly direction—and your spiritual connection or faith path. Your seed self, your *atman*, the true essence of your soul, has become occluded through the destructive patterns created by your obsession. It is time to investigate the power of turning over self-guidance to another.

Do you have a higher power? If so, do you rely on it/her/him?

Do you believe you don't have all the answers?

If you don't have a clear concept of a higher power, don't worry. Even the willingness to conceive of something, or someone, outside yourself that is capable of having solutions and concern for you is a start. If you are still resistant, pay particular attention to these additional questions.

What stands in your way of accepting guidance from something or someone outside yourself?

Is it a lack of trust? If so, in what way?

Is it difficulty in receiving help? If so, why?

Having an idea or a concept of a "power greater than" yourself will help you in the rest of your steps; however, this concept can change. Briefly record your current thoughts and feelings about a higher power, which you can refer to later.

The *yamas* and *niyamas*, or restraints and observances, respectively, mirror values that are present in recovery. In particular, yoga's observance of surrender, or *ishvara pranidhana,* is a useful practice in Step Two. Allow yourself to embrace the idea that there is a beneficent guide for your life.

Can you celebrate having a guide in your life?

When you have created, acknowledged, or affirmed a power greater than yourself, do you have an issue with the concept of being restored to sanity? Do you accept that behaviors related to your addiction were not a sane and healthy way—in mind, body, or spirit—to treat yourself or others?

Do you believe that you, in a more healthy frame of mind, would not have done, said, or thought many things you had while wrapped up in your addiction?

Finding bottom is a gift; a gift to move upward and outward. The root of your addiction, the source of your obsession, will give you the fertile ground for growth. All systems seek homeostasis, or the ability to obtain and maintain internal balance and equilibrium. When out of balance, you lose equanimity in your mental outlook, judgment, and wisdom as well as in your energy and physical layers. You may also fall out of connection with your higher power. You can use the model of the koshas to evaluate your health and sanity. Look at your layers and their state of *un*-health, or *dis*-ease, due to your addiction.

> *Physical layer:* How has your addiction impacted your body, immune system, digestion, other body functions/systems, etc.?

> *Energy layer:* How has your addiction impacted your vitality, breathing, and levels of energy?

Mental/emotional layer: How has your addiction impacted your ability to feel, to empathize, and find compassion and forgiveness? Can you identify any body sensations related to anxiety or fear?

Wisdom layer: How has your addiction impacted your ability to assess and choose or find and use your self-awareness?

Spiritual/bliss layer: How has your addiction impacted your ability to connect with the bliss of the universe and to all beings?

Once you understand your overall health, can you trust and believe you can be brought into balance in each of the five koshas?

The *gunas* are a paradigm you can use to see where you are stuck or ungrounded. The three states are *tamas* (heavy, stuck, and stagnant), *rajas* (movable, mobile, and frenetic), and *sattva* (content, harmonious, and stable).

In general, what has been your most prevalent state when you recall your active addiction and, perhaps, early recovery?

Let's return to the chakras, the energy centers in the body, looking at them from the point of view of Step Two: how your addiction has damaged them and how they can be restored to balance with the help of your higher power. You can better understand the impact of a chakra being over- or underactive when you understand what they provide when balanced.

Root chakra: This is the source of your security and sense of self. When in balance, it allows you to feel secure, to deal with life as it comes up, and to attend to the basics of everyday living, such as making your bed, keeping a tidy home, going to work, and paying your bills. When it is in balance, you feel rooted and grounded, aware of both supporting yourself and getting adequate support from others.

Do you feel grounded, emotionally settled, and secure in life?

Do you regularly attend to the mundane, daily aspects of your life?

Are you aware of your support systems?

Are you able to reach out to your support systems?

Sacral chakra: This energy center is where your feelings reside. While the root chakra seeks stability, the sacral chakra is healthy when it can move and doesn't get stuck. This is where you experience the forces of emotions, feelings, and desire. Your desire for pleasure is in the sacral energy center, and you may encounter your aliveness as well as your emotional identity here. This is also where your sense of sexuality resides. Becoming aware of how you feel is consciousness elevating. Your vitality increases when you connect your intimacy and integrity with your values and your physical body in an authentic way.

From a point of greater awareness, you can use the balance of the chakras to choose how you move and grow.

Are you aware of how you feel right now? Please describe.

Do you feel stuck in one emotion or another?

Can you tell if unbridled pleasure seeking has caused the sacral chakra to be over stimulated?

Solar plexus chakra: When in balance, this chakra aligns you with your competence, skills, and ability to cope with challenges. You gain inspiration from the throat, third eye, and crown chakras—your spiritual inputs—and you stay grounded with the energy from the root, sacral, solar plexus, and heart chakras. And, you may combine practice and intention in the solar plexus chakra, moving through the world with a clear sense of self-definition.

Do you feel in control or controlling? How does this show up in your life?

Have you lost a sense of direction in your life? If you answered yes, please describe.

Do you tend to get hot under the collar when you are challenged or do you become withdrawn? Please describe.

Do you feel that you've got this and don't need your higher power to assist you in recovery? Please describe.

Heart chakra: This is the region of your self-compassion and love. The heart chakra moves toward balance when you stop hurting yourself. You become aware of being at one with the universe, a part of all creation, when this energy center is in balance. Returning to sanity means to address and heal your sense of separateness and estrangement. Also the region of your social identity can be found in the heart chakra, growing beyond being alone toward being part of humanity.

Do you still feel terminally unique? In what ways?

Do you feel that others may handle recovery successfully, but you cannot? Give at least three examples.

Are you concerned that you are not able to return to sanity and are in some way broken? If answered yes, why do you feel this way?

Do you feel cut off from a higher power that you used to know? Or, do you feel you cannot connect to one at all? What is the reason you are unable to connect?

Throat chakra: You speak your truth from this space. The throat chakra is the transition from the lower chakras that concern themselves with grounding, pleasure, abilities, and connection to others with the insight and universal consciousness found in the remaining two chakras beyond the throat—the third eye and crown. You synthesize inspiration with worldly concerns and express yourself, your truth, with your voice and other modes of expression.

Do you feel choked off from the world? If yes, how does this show up in your life?

Do you feel choked off from your higher power? If yes, how does this show up in your life?

Are you able to trust your own voice and your thoughts? Why or why not?

Are you able to ask for help?

The throat chakra is also source of quiet listening. Are you able to listen to others? Are you able to discern wild talk from wise speech? How does the quality of quiet listening show up in your life?

Third eye chakra: This chakra expresses balanced energy around seeing and intuition: being able to see your goals and navigate toward them as well as discerning your internal intuition. Your dreams and visualizations, as well as being able to see the big picture, come from a healthy third eye chakra.

Is it hard to believe in a future where you would "turn it over"—whatever or whoever *it* is—to a higher power? Explain.

Do you feel that you can no longer trust your instincts and intuition? Why or why not?

Do you feel you have lost clarity when you look at your life in regards to your addiction? If yes, give at least three examples.

Can you tap into self-trust sufficiently to believe you can proceed in a healthy direction in your life? If not, what actions can you take to build trust?

Crown chakra: This is the space of your higher consciousness and an energy that links you to your higher power; think of it as a universal connection. (We will delve into the aspects and resources of the crown chakra in subsequent steps.) For now, consider your relationship with the possibility of having a higher power and finding your authentic self.

Do you continue to have difficulty in believing in a divine energy (or resource) that would care for you? If so, what actions can you take to help you find/believe in a loving higher power/divine energy?

Do you doubt that you can find and nurture your true self?

The ideas behind Step Two are hope, faith, open-mindedness, and clarity. Regardless of where you start or how you abandoned your ethics and values while under the influence of your addiction, *there is hope.* With willingness and open-mindedness, you can find clarity, which comes, in part, from giving up the reins and letting the grace of the universal consciousness—a higher power—guide you into health.

POSE

To embody the ideas of "turning it over" with both faith and hope, try Child's Pose, which is a comforting pose. You can curl over a bolster, a stack of pillows or a thick, folded blanket. You can curl up hips to heels, arms outstretched, forehead to the floor. While this is traditionally a prone pose with your face and chest toward the floor, you can also curl on your side or lay on your back with knees to chest. For more details, you can refer to Chapter Two of *Yogic Tools for Recovery* or follow the guidance provided in a short video at www.centralrecoverypress.com.

MEDITATION/VISUALIZATION PRACTICE

Read the following text all the way through and then, remembering as much as you can, prepare to enjoy a self-directed visualization. In yoga classes, as well as in life, we learn to take a break. Take a few moments to return to sanity before deciding, proceeding, and commencing with your day.

Either sitting or lying down, get comfortable. Bring attention to your breath. Bring your awareness to the inhale and the exhale, the rise and fall of your chest, and the swelling and softening of your belly. Do this eight or ten times. Do this until you experience release but not so much that you feel sleepy. Take your awareness away from your breath and move to your imagination. Imagine yourself in a place that is comforting to you: a field, a beach, a meadow. It could be a comfortable chair in a library or on a porch of a house that you make up or remember. If you are remembering a specific location, let it be some place where you have happy memories, playful thoughts, or sensations of being cared for.

Bring your attention to more and more details. What are the colors around you? What is the weather like? Is it morning or evening? Can you hear any sounds: birds, trees rustling, water, or waves? If you are indoors, what sounds can you hear? What is the room like? Remember this is your imagination, and you can create the space any way you want it to be.

Find a place of comfort and ease, where you feel well, secure, and at ease. Stay in the place as long as you like, and when you are ready to come back, just open your eyes.

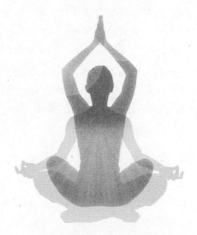

STEP THREE

We made a decision to turn our will and our lives
over to the care of God *as we understood Him.*

RECOVERY CONCEPTS

Faith, Willingness, Trust, Commitment

GUIDING YOGIC PRINCIPLE

"All things are created by the Om;
The love-form is His body. He is without form,
without quality, without decay:
Seek thou union with Him!"

KABIR

Continuing the concept of care that was started in the Second Step, you now look at turning your life over to the care of a higher power. Even if you have just started to discover a connection with your universal spirit, you can begin your companionship with this force. At this point, you have discovered some hope that you could be returned to sanity; now, you will proceed through the steps with this concept and let the outcome—the development of your healing—be in the hands of your higher power. It may seem as if this is just a deeper shade of believing that something could restore you—and it is, it is. It is the expansion of this type of care into the rest of your life. You not only can be returned to wellness, but this spiritual companion will also be there for you as you grow and develop in your recovery, one day at a time.

Follow spiritual guidance in respect to every decision. The Third Step invites you to consult with your spiritual guide at every significant juncture and decision in your day. This may sound like a lot, and at first it feels that way. A willingness to focus your life in a holistic and healthy direction—one that supports your recovery, needs, and actions—requires a guiding light. As you may have heard in meetings, "our best thinking got us here." It is time to be willing to let something else guide you.

The klesha of *ishvara pranidhana* can mean to devote oneself to a supreme or personal god. Practicing this observance may be seen as an all-inclusive Third Step. What would your supreme and personal higher power be like? What qualities would it/she/he have? What intentions, ethics, and values would this being or force embody?

What is standing in your way of being willing? What is difficult about turning your will and life over to the care of another?

Sometimes the challenge is letting go. You may think there is still something you can or should do. You may think you have got this and don't need to refer to your higher power.

Do you have difficulty letting go?

Do you have an idea why that is?

In order to turn your will and your life over the care of a guardian spirit, you might need to explore your concept of faith. What does faith mean to you?

The yama of *aparigraha*, non-attachment or non-greed, can be of some help during Step Three. If you are holding on to an outcome or an accolade (i.e., "You did it!"), you are not consulting your higher power. Or, you may be trying to avoid a painful result or holding on to the pleasure that something gives you, which relates to the kleshas of dvesha or raga.

> What if you have to give up something that you really like? What if you have to do something you don't like? What is standing in your way of letting go may be what you are holding on to.

> How do you consider pleasure, pain, attachment, and even greed as you look at your addiction and the unwillingness you may feel about turning over your life?

Svadhyaya is the niyama that is centered around the practice of self-study. Perhaps, there are lessons you learned as a youth that are no longer useful to you in regards to the idea of having a higher power, or someone who would be your consultant on life's journey.

> Do you recall any ideas about a higher power that stem from your childhood or young adulthood that are standing in your way now? Are there preconceptions that might benefit from re-examination?

The root and crown chakras are connected in the Third Step. The foundation, the fundamental idea of you being supported and grounded, rests in your root chakra. Your connection to your spiritual self, your higher power and guide, rests in your crown chakra.

Referring to the notes you made in Step Two about the root and crown chakras, what do you need in order to experience some healing and balancing, to feel your faith, and find willingness to continue your recovery journey?

What can you do to find equilibrium here? (Refer to chart in the Appendix for some suggestions for how to balance the chakras.)

Karma is the yoga of doing your work and leaving the rest alone. Step Three is the first of several steps that reminds you to do your work and leave the outcome to your higher power. The work in this step may feel nebulous in that it is a letting go of work rather than being engaged in an activity. When you turn your will and your life over to the care of a universal spirit, you let go of outcomes.

Right now, what are some issues that you are not comfortable letting go?

Taking a moment and going inward, discern what you feel as you contemplate letting go. What is your breath like? Can you express the feeling you have and where it is located in your body when you imagine letting go?

Anandamaya is your spiritual bliss layer. This is the part of your five koshas that is being reflected upon during the Third Step. You have the opportunity to revisit your relationship with your higher power: to develop it or to change it. This is a time to recognize the good that is within you. You will remain connected with the internal good as you look to connect with the good that exists outside you.

Notice how you feel when you consider this connection with the spirit that wishes to care for you. Are you able to discern a feeling, a sensation, or a thought of universal connection as you do Step Three? What does that look like for you?

POSE

The poses for Step Three have been chosen to open your heart. You can arrange yourself in a restorative yin, or cooling energy, pose or you can practice a yang, or more active, heart-opening, pose.

The yin pose could be lying on your back over a bolster or a blanket so that your chest is lifted, your head is supported, and your legs are either bent with your feet on the ground or extended with your heels on the ground. If you choose to do the Modified Lying Pose with Props, you can refer to the process in Chapter Three of *Yogic Tools for Recovery* or follow the guidance provided in a short video at www.centralrecoverypress.com.

The yang, or active pose, would be a crescent lunge, a Warrior I, or any pose with your fingers laced together and your arms raised or behind your back, lifting them behind you as you fold forward. (Refer to Poses to Align Your Chakras in the Appendix for some more options.)

MEDITATION

Prepare a space, a place to sit comfortably. Read the following text all the way through once before you begin. Don't be concerned if you don't remember it all. You will remember as much as you are supposed to. Set a timer for ten minutes, or more if you prefer.

Spend the first five breaths settling into your seated posture. Take five more breaths, noting the sounds in the room and beyond. With the next five breaths, consider the idea that the universe, your chosen higher power, your concept of other, cares deeply for you and wants the best for you. Visualize a place, a space where you can be content. Find a place of healing and security. Continue to imagine yourself there with the sensation of care, where you are not alone, in which you can find and have trust in your higher power.

Return to the present moment slowly and with care when the timer chimes.

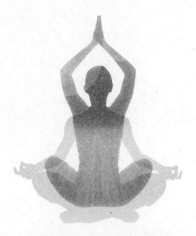

STEP FOUR

We made a searching and fearless
moral inventory of ourselves.

RECOVERY CONCEPTS

Courage, Review, Assessment

GUIDING YOGIC PRINCIPLE

"Through self-study comes union
with one's chosen deity."

SUTRA 2.44

The first three steps have grounded and prepared you for the journey of self-discovery. You are now ready to move into the first of the action steps. It is time to reaffirm your center, connect with your intention related to your recovery, and proceed.

Refer to your First Step and firmly visualize the behavior or substance you are now abstinent from. Recall the unmanageability and the *dis*-ease it had been causing in your life and throughout your body. The Fourth Step is where you dig down and look back to the nature, the expression, the characteristics, and the processes that you became accustomed to in your active addiction. Only by investigation can you begin to make choices about how to participate in the changes that are needed in your life.

The first three steps are strongly aligned with the first two chakras—the root and sacral—and the crown chakra. It is important to bring them in balance, so they can provide you with the support you need as you continue your investigation. You will get to know more about the kleshas, the yamas, the niyamas, and all the other concepts, too, as you understand how deeply you were impacted by your addiction. Before you continue with the steps, take some time to bring awareness to the root, the sacral, and the crown chakras.

MEDITATION

A recording of this mediation is available at www.centralrecoverypress.com.

Find a comfortable way to sit. Breathe in and out. Set an intention to bring your attention to the inner landscape of your body. This inner world is where chakras of your being can be found. This is where your connection between inner being and the outer world meet. This is where heaven and Earth come together within you. This union of inner and outer is unique to you. The concept of union is universal. Going inward in this manner is a way for you to honor that uniqueness, the individual and precious being that you are. It is also a way to connect with the universal and discover how you are related to everything and everyone. You are strong and have a curiosity that wants to explore your own inner workings. Let yourself prepare for the journey of this meditation without judgment and with curiosity. Pull attention from the outer world and into the inner world.

Begin this investigation with your earthly concerns. Bring your attention to the everyday aspects of your life—the regular sustaining activities, such as bed making and doing dishes, and the personal preparations for the day, such as wearing clean clothes and eating a nourishing breakfast. Also, look at the touch points of sanity you are building in your life, engaging in morning readings and meditation as you reflect on your day with awareness and non-attachment. You may recall your plans for getting together with others at a meeting or with your sponsor. Be supportive of yourself and your recovery and be with others who support you and your recovery.

The symbol of the root chakra is the earth. You can use this image as your resource: how you engage in life, what type of "soil" and nurturing earth you look to ground in, and how you plant yourself through your own footwork to find your foundation. Once you find this space, you root, ground, and plant yourself to prepare to grow into your new life journey. Pause now and reflect on your root, your grounding. The focus of the root chakra is self-preservation; you once thought this was available only through your addictive actions, but you found this road would lead to *dis*-ease, injury, madness, or death. You can find self-preservation in recovery. With respectful actions in everyday life and surrounding yourself with people who have solid recovery, you can find support for your recovery.

Breathe in and out with that sense of planting yourself firmly into the ground and rising out and up from your foundation into the fullness of your own being.

The second chakra is the sacral chakra. The element, or symbol, of the sacral chakra is water, which is a moving and mobile quality. When you turn your life over to the care of your universal spirit, you prepare yourself to take action in your recovery. While this energy center is oriented toward pleasure and away from pain or difficulty, you now are learning to reframe what true, ethical pleasure is and how it can heal and support self-esteem rather than denigrate it. You may discover how discomfort can be a tool for growth.

In the sacral chakra, you follow the flow toward healing activities, such as cleaning out the closet of your life, keeping what fits and suits you now, and letting go of the rest. Using the sensations you find in your body as you consider the faith, trust, and hope that you have developed doing your first three steps, you are now strong enough to consider the emotional and behavioral impacts of active addiction. The sacral energy center is important as it signals positive and negative feelings. As you mindfully move toward the calm, harmonious, yet complex feelings of recovery, you can still be aware of the sharp and possibly difficult feelings that memories bring you. Returning to your grounded nature allows you to look at your life in safety and note the feelings that arise as you do the Fourth Step.

Through your second chakra, you open to the flow of feelings, the waters of emotions, an awareness of your senses. You open to feelings and emotions as well as to your senses of sexuality and intimacy. You begin to investigate these qualities as they relate to closeness with another person. You also begin to balance the polarities of the soul—left/right, in/out, up/down. By balancing these polarities, you begin to embody unity in your core. You have the right to feel, and you can let go of feelings of guilt. Guilt will block your healing.

Let your awareness and your breath sit still here, in the space between your hip bones, letting go of judgment as feelings come and go. Avoid judgment—that sense of right and wrong—and know the space in between where all possibilities exist. You are whole.

Moving now to the seventh chakra—the crown—it is useful to recognize that you are not alone. All your sufferings, our sufferings, have been noted through the ages. We are connected to one another. You are connected through your journey in recovery by way of the steps and your connection with the paths of others in their journey to freedom through waking up. That is why the steps have been written and what the sages and wise people of yoga have documented for us. You are not alone.

As you move toward connection with others, you also practice letting go, non-attachment, letting go of the way things were. Using your connection to your higher power, you are given the strength you need to look at your life, choosing what you keep and determining what you need to learn from the past. As you do this you may discover that you no longer have to repeat unuseful and damaging behaviors. Connecting again to the root chakra, bloom up through the crown chakra, being aware as you do so, doing what you can, and leaving the outcome, the result, in the hands of your higher power. Move through the seven chakras releasing what no longer serves you; the timing and result are in the hands of your higher power.

Take a few more breaths, open your eyes, and orient yourself in the room.

ASANA PRACTICE

If you find you are feeling anxious, fearful, or have the desire to procrastinate, there are a few practices you can do to get yourself centered and ready to work. You can try one, or all, not as tools of delay but to prepare yourself in the best way possible to do the deep work you have before you.

There are both yin and yang practices—sedate and active, respectively—that can prepare you for the Fourth Step. You can start with yang and end with yin, do one of each, or try only one pose; it's your choice. Using the Poses to Align Your Chakras chart in the Appendix, select poses from the root, sacral, and crown chakra offerings. You can also select poses that feel good to you, concentrating on the connections to the ground and the movement of the breath in the pauses between the poses. Notice how you feel going into the poses *and* coming out of them.

BREATH PRACTICE

Ujjayi breath is a strengthening and calming breathing process done by exhaling slowly through a partially closed throat—sometimes described as sounding like an ocean. Use a slow ujjayi breath to provide calm and grounding before you begin Step Four.

SENSE THERAPIES

You can listen to music before you begin or as you work on Step Four. Be sure it is calming and affirming rather than stimulating. You may have a diffuser or scented candle with a bright smell to keep you focused (cinnamon, citrus, or rosemary). Prepare your space so that it is simple and uncluttered. Be comfortable but avoid sleepiness. Eat lightly and be sure you pause to nourish yourself when needed, and avoid distracting yourself with constant replenishment of things to eat or drink. You are now ready to begin.

The Fourth Step asks you to review your moral inventory, directing you to the practice of self-study, or *svadhyaya*, which is one of the niyamas. Step Four also directs you to use materials outside yourself to make this evaluation. Read sacred texts; listen to others; go to houses of worship and recovery meetings. These can help lead you to learn more about what it means to become the best person you aspire to be.

With this lens of wise teachings and words from others, you learn more about who you are and how you want to be. This information can also be used to evaluate the missteps of the past. Affirming and reaffirming your recovery morals (values) can help you discover where you left them behind or ignored them in your past.

Use compassion as you wander the landscape of past behaviors. Avoid looking at your past as a mine field and more as a field to be mined for clues to how your past behavior conflicted with your ethics and values. Discover how addiction and obsession directed you away from what you now feel is your true self.

Be kind and be comprehensive. Do not cheat yourself out of this amazing experience by avoiding difficulty or pain. Use tools to help you through and be thorough. This is not your first time through the steps, so you may have some memory of both the difficulties and the gifts of this process.

Using self-study to determine what your values and beliefs are, think back to those rooms and places of worship or discussion that you revere. What have you heard and agreed with at meetings and with your sponsor or friends? What do you believe? Asking yourself these questions is a good place to start; you can refer to these answers as you continue forward. Looking back, remember what your experience was like and what your intention for your life is now.

Consider using the yamas and the niyamas as you evaluate your current understanding of your ethics and values. The yamas, or restraints, are classified as non-harming, non-lying, non-stealing, non-excess, and non-attachment. The niyamas, or observances, are known as cleanliness, contentment, self-study, discipline, and surrender.

My values in respect to my relationships with others are

My values in respect to my work/job/career are

My values in respect to my health and well-being are

My values in respect to my financial well-being are

My values in respect to myself and my boundaries are

List other values, if any, that you have not yet listed.

Use this information about your values as you consider the impacts of your addiction. Then, think about the koshas and note how the nature of your behavior in active addiction impacted you: your body, your energy, your impressions and emotions, your intellect, and your spiritual being and connection.

How did your behavior in active addiction impact your physical ability?

How did your behavior in active addiction impact your energy?

How did your behavior in active addiction impact your emotions and how you interpreted the world around you?

How did your behavior in active addiction impact your intellect, judgment, and character?

How did your behavior in active addiction impact your spirituality?

Keeping in mind the issue(s) and addiction you wrote about in your First Step, explain how your actions, attitudes, and behaviors were influenced by your sources of mental torment, or sufferings, known as the kleshas.

What false understanding or erroneous thinking did you have?

What was the result or impact of this false perception or misunderstanding?

What role did aversion play in your behavior?

Can you determine the types of craving, attachment, or longing that influenced your behavior?

There are a few ways the ego, or asmita, can drive you. You may feel you are worth nothing or you may experience a self-centered ego that believes no one else matters. Or, you may experience them both.

How was your ego involved in the choices you made and the actions you took in active addiction?

Abhinivesha is the fear of change, transformation, or even death. You may act in certain unskilled ways when faced with uncertain or change. And, you can often fall into old behavior patterns.

How have your actions and choices been influenced by abhinivesha?

Reflect back to your chakras. Can you determine which of your chakras were either over- or underactive and thus influenced your behavior? Or, conversely, which of your behaviors caused a chakra to become either over- or underactive? Refer to How Chakras Affect Your Body in the Appendix to remind yourself of the out-of-balance conditions and properties.

• Root chakra

• Sacral chakra

• Solar plexus chakra

• Heart chakra

- Throat chakra

- Third eye chakra

- Crown chakra

Notice that the previous series of questions, as well as your work so far, have been an examination and investigation of how you felt and acted while in active addiction. You were not asked about what others have done nor were you asked to name other people who were involved. You were asked to go inside yourself. The purpose of this Fourth Step—perhaps a little different from the original intention—is that you journey inward to see how *you* are doing, feeling, processing life, and learning from your choices and decisions. You can even determine where your choices and decisions stem from so that the next time you meet similar challenges you have more options.

Please do not skip this part of your fourth-step work: Intentionally look toward the good, the ethical, and the comfortable. Experience those aspects of yourself that give you a sense of wholeness. Now, review the work you have just completed using this sense of self. You may be pleasantly surprised. You may find events and sensations that were pleasurable, fun, or humorous. You may find pockets of ease that are tension free. You are not all good or all bad. A thorough inventory looks at all aspects. This is an opportunity to notice how your true self was trying to be heard. This, too, is part of your inventory.

Note instances of care and concern, loving kindness, or fairness. Scan your five layers of being for memories and events that allowed you to feel complete, more yourself. Use the model of the chakras to recall moments when you felt a balanced connection to those energy centers.

Were there times when you were able to let go, face adversity, find courage, and be content? Let yourself be still and recall. Write down as many as you can now.

Take some time now to read over what you have written. Pause and take it all in. Breathe. Before moving to Step Five, look over this vital material and see if you can discern any patterns.

Are there any issues or processes that pop up repeatedly? Is there a theme? Make some notes here about your self-reflection.

In the next step, you will share your fourth-step work with a trusted person. You see what you see now; and with guidance and compassion, you may see more. This is the path to self-awareness, realization, and healing. You have done a good job.

BREATH AND BODY-SENSE AWARENESS

As you conclude Step Four, take a moment to check in with your breath. Check in with your internal landscape and the feelings in your body—your jaw, your heart rate, your chest, your belly, and your legs. Are your arms or legs becoming tense? Is your jaw gripping? You may feel ill at ease or discomfort in belly or in your gut. Where else may you be having physical signs? Check in often as you work. Your body will give you information that your mind may gloss over. Feel your body and believe it.

POSE

You have been looking inward. The calming nature of a forward fold can sustain and refresh you. The forward fold can be done from a standing position or seated on the floor. Step Four is not a time to overreach, stressing and straining the body for an ideal forward fold. If you choose to do the Supported Forward Fold pose, you can refer to the process in Chapter Four of *Yogic Tools for Recovery* or follow the guidance provided in a short video at www.centralrecoverypress.com. Experiment with the pose and find the posture that sustains you.

PRANAYAMA

To cleanse and release any trapped emotions, you can try a bellows breath, or *bhastrika*. This is a practice of enforced exhale with a full, intentional, natural inhale. The inhale and exhale should be of equal force. You determine a number of repetitions—perhaps start with ten—and commit to sustaining that number. Follow with a period of rest. Repeat for a total of three sets. (**Note:** Do not practice bellows breath if you're pregnant or have uncontrolled hypertension, epilepsy, seizures, or panic disorder. You should also avoid practicing bellows breath on a full stomach, so please wait at least two hours after eating.)

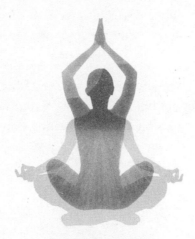

STEP FIVE

We admitted to God, to ourselves, and to another
human being the exact nature of our wrongs.

RECOVERY CONCEPTS

Integrity, Trust, Commitment

GUIDING YOGIC PRINCIPLE

"The mind becomes tranquil through the practice of friendliness
toward the happy, compassion toward the miserable,
joy toward the virtuous, and equanimity toward the non-virtuous."

SUTRA 1.33

This is the time to practice self-care. This is the time to reaffirm your goals and reassure yourself. Step Five doesn't have to be a scary event. In fact, you may have been sharing your Fourth Step with your sponsor all along. Certainly a degree of prayer and meditation have been practiced as well. Your higher power knows your past, your journey, and your purpose.

This time with your sponsor may be a ceremonial event honoring the conclusion of an intense process. You two may spend some time talking about what this work was like for you, or you may remind one another of important points or aspects of your investigation. In any case, this is a significant transition from delving into the past to evaluating how the wrongs of your past can or have influenced your present, and the themes of your choices and feelings may now be apparent.

POSE AND BREATH PRACTICE

To prepare for Step Five, move your body in a yoga pose sequence, something with a little more enthusiasm than slow moving yin, or restorative, poses. Or, you can choose a breath practice that is both cleansing and brightening. For a yoga pose sequence, use something such as the 100 Breaths before Breakfast or a simple slow Warrior II series, which can be found by doing a online search.

For a breath sequence, consider bellows breath, which allows for forceful exhales followed by strong inhales in a sequence of twenty or more in a row. This quantity of breaths is a little more than you practiced in the prior step, so if it feels like too many, drop back to a number of repetitions that makes you comfortable. Repeat two more times, resting after each set of breaths and bringing your awareness to how you feel. The strong flow of movements or the dedicated breath practice will clear your mind and remove excess anxiety that may occur before sharing with your sponsor or reading your whole Fourth Step in one sitting.

During the Fifth Step, you need to be strong and open to sharing. Some poses that can strengthen your back and open your heart are Sphinx pose, Cobra pose, or any Locust variation. If you choose to do the Supported Sphinx pose, you can refer to the process in Chapter Five of *Yogic Tools for Recovery* or follow the guidance provided in a short video at www.centralrecoverypress.com. While poses like this look simple, you may find that, like the steps, they are simple but not easy. Choose one or a few and do them now.

Now, you have prepared. You are ready to share your Fourth Step. You have done good work. Trust the process. As Sutra 1.1 states, "Here follows instruction in union."

It is time to begin learning from the work you have done. In this next series of questions, you are looking to ground yourself in preparation for your discussion. A way to take a quick, internal inventory is to consider how you feel at the level of all your koshas. Breathe in and out a few times before reading each question in this section to see how you are doing.

What is the status of your physical layer? Did you sleep well last night? Have you eaten wisely? Well? Recently? Sufficient? Too much? Have you moved around today? Do you have stuck energy?

How is your energy layer? Are you vibrating with the feeling of being anxious? Do you feel in the doldrums, perhaps dulling your feelings? There is no right way to feel—just notice how you are doing.

How are you processing your feelings? Are you excited in anticipation, or is there sadness? Are you anticipating shame or guilt? Are you feeling disconnected from your feelings or overengaged? Notice what your emotional layer is telling you.

Are you perhaps intellectualizing the process? Do you already have an idea about how this sharing will proceed? Do you have expectations or assumptions? Is reason overwhelming how you feel? Are you open to whatever happens? No single thought or pattern may sit still in your mind; you may meander through many thoughts. Take a moment to "photograph" what is in your mind right now and write it down.

To continue preparation for sharing your Fourth Step with your trusted person, take a moment to connect with your higher power, your universal spirit. Perhaps, take a moment to find that spirit in you with the knowledge that you are unfolding and revealing it in this fifth-step process.

Another tool for checking in with yourself before discussing your Fourth Step is to connect with your chakras. Get grounded and do things that allow you to feel secure and connected. Be sure you have sufficient energy for sharing. Do something that will give you a sense of how in balance your root chakra is. Check in with your sacral chakra, making sure you are not too moveable or *rajasic* but remaining open to solutions as you hear yourself speak. Are you ready to experience the closeness that this type of intimacy requires?

The solar plexus chakra will give you a sense of personal choice, mastery, and appropriate power. Your heart can open to compassion for yourself and your journey—the path that got you here. You will need to be in touch with your throat chakra. Your ability to merge the mundane, daily attributes of the first four chakras with the intuitive and spiritual connections from your sixth and seventh chakras is critical. Take time to speak, hum, or sing; find your voice. Also, be prepared to listen, to really hear, what is being shared with you when you do your Fifth Step. How does your throat feel? Do you feel that you are able to discern between the real and the unreal? Are you open to your intuition and your self-understanding? A balanced third eye chakra will help with that.

Finally, take a moment to truly release yourself into the loving arms of your spiritual guide, your higher power. See if you can connect strongly in trust with your spiritual self. Allow the possibility that you are going to learn exactly what you need to learn from this process.

Check in with your seven chakras and make some notes about what you found.

You are sharing your Fifth Step with your listening self, your inquisitive and nonjudgmental self. You are sharing this with your spirit side, your higher power directly. Take a moment to hold that concept and make your Fourth Step an offering, a prayer, and a blessing. You are also sharing with your sponsor. Let that be a grace as well.

Once you have completed your process with your sponsor, take time to savor your tenacity, willingness, and integrity. As you prepared for this session with your sponsor, you began with yoga or pranayama, and now you may want to restore yourself afterward with some self-care.

This investigation and sharing is hard work. It is also an opportunity to practice healthy rewards after a job well done. Take a walk or a hike; listen to or play music; practice meditation or yin yoga or any other sense therapy. These activities are useful after this kind of deep work. You may schedule a massage or take a luxurious bath with scented Epsom salts or candles. Eat well. While cake may be a part of a celebratory meal, this isn't the time to reward yourself with something you feel is not healthy for you. It could be cake, but it could also be any of a number of other foods. Choose wisely and you will feel good all the way through. Then take time to rest.

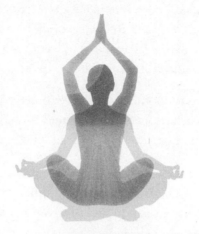

STEP SIX

We were entirely ready to have God
remove all these defects of character.

RECOVERY CONCEPT

Willingness, Intention

GUIDING YOGIC PRINCIPLE

"Practice becomes fully grounded when continued
for a long time with devotion and right action."

SUTRA 1.14

Letting go of character defects sounds like an easy decision to make. Who wouldn't want to be free of defects? On the other hand, you might have noticed in your Fourth Step that there were fears, pain, insecurity, and tender emotions that were being protected by defects. Each of these tender, perhaps negative emotions seemed to have a role in keeping the true you deep inside, keeping you safe, free from the dangers of being seen. Each one of us has a unique constellation of these defects. Look through your Fourth Step and see if you can begin to list your defects.

We all have commonalities with one another in what we protected in our active addiction. What is your constellation of actions and behaviors? What were they providing you? How will you get your needs met, your emotions protected, and your fear abated if these are gone?

What would happen if you didn't yell when you were angry? Would the other person know how you felt? How can you become included in activities with others without resorting to manipulative behavior? How can you get what you need without being needy? How would you feel if you completed your duties, tasks, or assignments rather than putting them off? Would you have to keep working at it and redo or edit it? Would you fall into the grips of perfectionism? How would you protect yourself from possible future pain if you didn't guard yourself with resentment? How would you look at and appreciate your life if you stopped being jealous or envious? Would you take steps to change your life? If the agitation of dissatisfaction went away, how would you feel energized? And so on through the list of character defects that you have created.

When contemplating change, it is best if you are rested and grounded. It is hard to be willing to let go of what has partially served you in the past if you are feeling unmoored or vulnerable. There are a few ways to find stability and tap into your inner strength; hatha yoga practice is one way to find that strength. Whether you do an active practice—moving from pose to pose through a sequence, pausing for only a breath or two in each posture—or if you do a slower practice, you can use the time in motion to rest your brain and let the ideas fall from your head into your heart as feelings.

You can contemplate willingness and consider letting go of unwanted traits completely as you practice your postures. Avoid holding onto a specific result, a sequence of release of the defects, or any active intention as you hold each pose. Sun Salutation, done slowly or in the active style, is one way to move in a wholesome way.

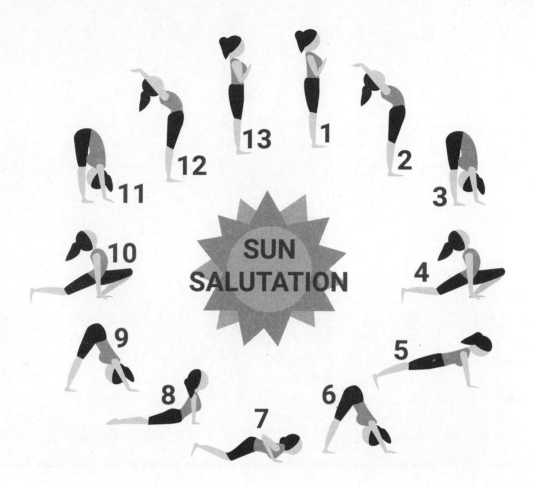

SUN
SALUTATION

Following the sequence, lie in *savasana,* also called Tranquility pose, for at least five minutes. Return to a seated position and continue your work on Step Six. Using the Fourth Step as a starting point, look at what you have discovered. You can mine a lot of information from your inventory, discovering behaviors you developed to defend yourself as well as to be defensive. There are attributes, actions, and attitudes that you developed to preserve your emotional safety, perhaps to protect your physical safety and defend your addiction, too. These no longer serve you as you move toward recovery and into a life of deeper integration. Step Six is a preparatory step. While the mind may rush to the results of being clear of characteristics that can be destructive to ourselves, our relationships, and our progress, the Sixth Step asks you to pause and ready yourself.

What are you ready to be relieved of? What impedes you from having a life where you are able to experience being happy, joyous, and free? Using the yogic tools you have been practicing, the following series of questions will allow you to explore what stands in your way of being your true self fully. Consider some defects you may have and what defensive behaviors you have developed. There may be two different lists, or they may converge. Don't worry too much about where your obstacles land; just start writing them down.

Consider the yamas as you look at your defects. Did you intentionally or unintentionally harm anyone or anything? Did you lie or steal? Do you have an issue with excess or with unhealthy attachments that verged on possessiveness?

Does any of your defensive behavior reflect the following obstacles: aversion or avoidance; craving or attachment; ego and a misunderstanding of yourself; or general fear of change, aging, or death? What stems from ignorance or false perceptions? How do you act when faced with these obstacles?

Do any of your defects or defenses arise when you are hungry, angry, lonely, or tired (i.e., HALT)? Can you relate certain behaviors with any of these conditions? Recall the five koshas, particularly the first four (the physical, energetic, mental/emotional, and intellectual layers), and write down any actions or behaviors you have when you are not in balance with HALT.

POSE

If you choose to do the Crocodile pose for Step Six, you can refer to the process in Chapter Six of *Yogic Tools for Recovery* or follow the guidance provided in a short video at www.centralrecoverypress.com.

MEDITATION

To set the stage of willingness in Step Six and to prepare for Step Seven, a period of meditation can help open your heart for change, the type of change that you yourself do not direct, the one that comes about when you are willing.

Use the chakras to see if there is any residual resistance to having your defects removed. Then prepare to meditate for ten minutes. Read the following text all the way through once before you begin, recalling as much as you can. There is no perfect here, no good or bad, right or wrong. Scan your body sensations. Sit quietly for a few moments. Breathe in and out. Again. Beginning at the base of your body, scan up through your legs, torso, neck, and head. Take a moment to take stock of how you feel right now. Do you sense any areas of tightness? Are there areas of neutrality or even comfort? Note these. Breathe again with attention.

Starting with the root chakra, how do you feel? Content, grounded, secure? Do you feel lethargic or do you have scattered thinking?

—Pause and reflect without judgment—

Bring your awareness a little higher, focusing on the area in between your hips. The sacral chakra is the seat of your fluid emotions. Can you connect with your feelings? Are you having difficulty letting go? Just see. Investigate. No reason to do anything at this moment. Just note it. Breathe into this awareness.

—Pause—

The solar plexus is the region of your self-respect and self-esteem. What do you feel here? Be aware of any information given to you in the form of a sensation in your "belly brain." Is there any sense of wanting to be perfect or wanting to do things perfectly? Is there concern about criticism from self or others? Breathe into the awareness.

—Pause—

Move your focus to the middle of your chest, into the middle of your body, your heart chakra. Breathe. Notice if there is any tightness or feeling of obstruction. Can you soften your body around your heart chakra? Can you sense compassion and forgiveness? Do you feel sad or self-pity? Are you denying your needs or experiencing a loss of boundaries? This work is hard.

—Pause and check in fully with how you are feeling—body, mind, and spirit—

We speak honestly and listen astutely from the throat chakra. This is the source of your positive energy and potential for growth. Is your throat open, the muscle loose and flexible? Do you feel a tightness or thickness in your neck? Are you holding back, based on some historical fear? Or, do you feel a rush of wanting to pour it all out, perhaps taking responsibility for everything? What is your truth?

—Stay here for several breaths—

When you move up to the third eye chakra, recall the gifts of balance: clear vision, understanding of the inner self, and being able to discern between truth and fiction. If you have had difficulties seeing the patterns of your defects and their associated fear, impulses, or desires, pause now. Recall willingness and imagine an open hand. Your "defences of character" are in your palm. Let your universal spirit choose.

—Breathe and pause—

Being open to your divine spirit and your higher power can emanate from your crown chakra. That is the gift here. If you are feeling overly intellectual or skeptical about this step and this process, these may be signs that your crown chakra is not in balance. Take breaths here and allow *no thought* to be your thought. This can be found in seeing thoughts and letting them go rather than not thinking at all. Breathe and let go. Rejoice in willingness.

—Pause, breathe, and, when you are ready, open your eyes—

With willingness fully in place, you can move on to the Seventh Step.

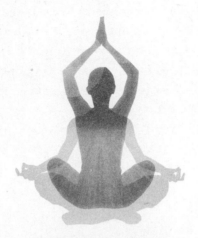

STEP SEVEN

We humbly asked Him to remove our shortcomings.

RECOVERY CONCEPTS

Humility, Readiness to Change

GUIDING YOGIC PRINCIPLE

"When the mind can distinguish between the causes of suffering
and the results, the cycle of suffering can be reduced."

SUTRA 4.30

How can yoga help with humility and the ability to ask for help? Yoga teaches us to be the right size, to be in our body, mind, and spirit as it is right now. The present moment is indeed the present, or gift, in yoga as it is in recovery. Another deeper aspect of yoga is understanding that life is not binary: There is no one way, no one right way and one wrong way. There are not good feelings and bad feelings, right emotions and wrong emotions. In other words, "It is what it is." If we think in terms of our shortcomings, defects, and defenses, this means having distinct emotional characteristics is not the issue, but rather it is our response to them, how we cling or avoid, and how we demonstrate them in the world.

Consider what being *the right size* means. How can you avoid comparing yourself to someone else (in yoga class, at work, at home, or in social media)?

How can you practice acceptance of your list of defects, i.e., seeing things clearly as they are?

How can you see yourself as no better and no worse than another being?

How can you accept yourself as being human?

Is it possible to avoid being either the victor or the martyr? What does this look like in your life?

What does *humility* mean to you?

Using their imagination, some people put their defects in the palm of their hand and let their higher power choose among them. Look inside yourself and honestly determine if you have a preference as to which defect or shortcoming goes first. Without judgment, become aware of preference. What has happened to me is that I hope for one of them, *my* choice, to be selected. It works best, however, if I turn over the whole batch.

I have experienced a great variety of shortcomings over the years. Among them have been expectation, overwork, underwork, anger, fear, control, neediness, and insecurity. My practice has been to write the defects on slips of paper, put the papers in my hand, and imagine that my universal spirit would choose one, open it, and give me enough challenge in this area so that I could improve my relationship with this shortcoming. The day will expose which one is actually the issue being addressed; often it is not the one I had hoped for.

What shortcomings would you write down today?

Do you find yourself having a preference about which one should be addressed first? Why?

As you ask for help, notice if you have some preference or idea about what kind of help you need. That could be part of your challenge. Or, it may be a defect: your desire to control or know what is best for you. It may be as if you knew which one was impeding you the most, which one was preventing you from being the most available to do the best service as you move through life. Perhaps, indeed, you don't. Allow your experience in doing better reveal the shortcoming that is ready to be removed. Do your best. Letting your intention be your most authentic and best self is all you can do.

The kleshas can provide a paradigm for looking at both the humility and the asking aspect of the Seventh Step. False understanding, the ego, grasping and craving, aversion and avoidance, and even fear of death can become lenses to look at humility and letting your higher power take charge of your defect removal.

How has ignorance or false understanding influenced your humility and ability to let your higher power choose which defect to remove?

Has grasping or craving had the same effect? What do you think you cannot live without? Are you still holding onto anger or resentment to keep you safe or insulated?

How about aversion or avoidance? Will it be too difficult or will there be other work to do if you address this shortcoming? Describe what this might look like.

Describe any aspects of your ego that stand in the way? What would your life look like if you let these go?

What defects do you fear losing that you have come to rely on? Describe how you rely on or use these defects.

POSE

If you choose to do the Reclined Twist pose, you can refer to the process in Chapter Seven of *Yogic Tools for Recovery* or follow the guidance provided in a short video at www.centralrecoverypress.com.

MEDITATION

Take a moment, once again, to refer to your First Step and your Fourth Step. Reaffirm your intention in doing the steps. This can be a moment to rekindle the purpose of your work and focus again on the *why* of what you are doing.

Bring your attention to the first three chakras: root, sacral, and solar plexus. These need to be in a state of balance—momentary, perhaps, but secure for now—so that the heart is open in willingness. Let's begin with an open-door meditation. Read the following text all the way through once before you begin. Then practice what you remember. Don't worry about the wording; the images you discover are the important thing. You could also have a friend read to you.

Get into your comfortable seated position for meditation. Notice the sounds around you. Let go of their purpose or meaning; accept that right now they have nothing to do with you and you have nothing to do with them. Imagine sounds as waves—merely a movement of molecules impacting your ears. Bring your attention to your physical sensations. Is there a hair on your cheek you need to brush away? Is there any part of your clothing that needs adjustment? Is your seated posture one you can maintain for a length of time? Attend to these distractions and then let them go. Be aware of your breath. Inhale, pause, exhale, and pause so that each part is of an equal length. Try this cycle for five to ten times.

—Pause—

Let go of conscious breathing and breathe in a comfortable way. Bring the soft focus of your closed eyes up to the level of your eyebrows, not uplifted with force but with a soft upward gaze. Then imagine looking out toward the horizon. Continue to breathe in a soft, slow manner.

—Pause—

You are approaching a door or a gate. The door could be to a home, a castle, a room, or some place you have never been before but seems friendly and new. You may imagine a gate in a hedge or fence that opens to a garden or meadow, a large yard you have never explored. You may be passing through some bushes on the bank of a stream or at the beach next to a lake or the ocean. In all these choices, you are opening a door or gate moving into a space that has the feeling of newness and pleasure.

—Pause—

Reach out and open the door or gate. Notice the quality of light as you swing it open. Look forward in curiosity.

—Pause—

What do you see? Look around and discover as much detail as possible.

—Pause—

Walk in, wander around, and take in the scenery, the objects, and the plants. Take in the amazing beauty around you.

—Pause—

Slip off your shoes and feel the ground. What texture is there? Find lush comfort under your feet. As you wander around, you notice a bench, stool, or a place on the ground that offers comfort for you to sit.

—Pause—

Take a seat and rest here. Let the beauty and space of this place fill your heart. Perhaps feelings well up—curiosity or comfort, the emotional tug of a memory, or the excitement of a new future. Find refuge in this new territory, one that has shed the trappings of the past and is open to the new, the previously unknown.

—Pause—

Sit and breathe in this new space that requires none of the old guards or defenses; it needs only care and wisdom to maintain its beauty. Continue to look around and discover more about this place: sounds, temperature, perhaps an animal or pet, and whatever gives you joy and connection. Breathe.

—Pause—

When you are ready, rise up. Either gather your shoes or slip them on. Turning slowly, move back toward the gate or door. Shut it behind you with the knowledge that this sweet space, this home or room, shore or meadow, is always here when you want it. Take some time to return to your awareness of the room or space you are seated in, and how your body is feeling. Then open your eyes.

Consider that the purpose of Step Seven is to remind you that the removal of your shortcomings develops you so that you can be of maximum service to others who are struggling. This includes yourself and those around you. However, you may not be the best person to discern which shortcomings are to be removed in order to do that.

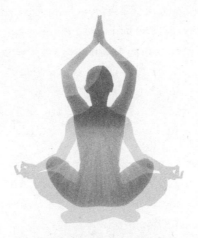

STEP EIGHT

We made a list of all persons we had harmed,
and became willing to make amends to them all.

RECOVERY PRINCIPLE

Empathy, Forgiveness, Responsibility

GUIDING YOGIC PRINCIPLE

"When disturbed by negative thoughts
cultivate positive thoughts."

SUTRA 2.33

Be kind, be still, and consider the purpose of Step Eight. In it's basic form, this step asks you to prepare a list and become willing—that's it. Try to avoid jumping ahead to Step Nine. In order to make your list, you will need to look back at your previous steps, particularly Step Four and possibly Step Five. Now is the time to consider others, the people who may have played a part in your actions and reactions. With full attention to the nature of your actions—without rationalization, defending, or justifying—prepare to list the names of the people involved. You may or may not make direct amends to these people. The present is not the time to think about that; just write down their names. Look inside and discover or remind yourself of your values, ethics, and current life in recovery. Would you have treated people in that way now?

Making amends sometimes means to apologize; other times, it means to change your relationships and approaches; and in other circumstances, it will mean both. Amends, or the changes you make in recovery, come from deep down inside, your true inner self, your atman. You are being transformed into, or perhaps returned to, your true nature.

Like the psychic change referenced in twelve-step literature, yoga wisdom has a lot to offer in regards to psychic changes. In fact, that is another thing that yoga and recovery share: developing a new way of life.

In a discussion about the niyamas, or the observances, Gary Kissiah, author and yogi, had this to say, which can help you as you prepare to make amends.

> Let's consider the use of *pratipaksa* [meeting thought and emotion with its opposite] in this situation. We can cultivate an opposing emotion, feeling, or energy. Why not visualize approaching this person with mental images of kindness, compassion, and peace? Why not imagine a positive interaction or a successful conversation?

While creating your list, you will examine who or what you took unwise action toward and then look toward replacing that unwise action with wise action. In Steps Six and Seven, you concretely and explicitly investigated your shortcomings and defensive actions. Also, you became ready to have them modified or removed or taught to exhibit those emotions or behaviors in a more mature and thoughtful way.

Before putting pen to paper, practice a little yoga, such as a Warrior Pose series. Or, you can practice meditation. The yoga practice reminds you of your hidden strength. The meditation introduces you to your new self, the person you are becoming as you practice your innermost ethics and ideals.

MEDITATION

If you choose to meditate, try this metta meditation. This is a set form of meditation also called *loving kindness*. You repeat words or phrases several times as you bring to mind people from your life. It is designed to help you soften your heart. The phrase you will be repeating is this: "May you be safe, may you be healthy, may you be happy. May you meet with ease of heart whatever comes your way in life." You can use these phrases of loving kindness, remembering as much of them as you can, or you can use other sentences to convey good wishes.

Sit and first bring to mind yourself, your heartfelt true self.
Repeat the phrases three times with honesty and compassion.

Next, bring to mind a person who has been helpful to you, a teacher, guide, or mentor. Center on one person at a time with fixed mental gaze and repeat the phrases three or more times.

Now, bring to mind someone who is neutral, someone you recognize but don't know well. It could be someone from work, the store, a meeting you attend, or a yoga class you go to. Bring his or her face to mind and repeat the phrases three times.

Bring to mind a difficult person, perhaps someone you are thinking of putting on your list. Bring his or her image firmly on the screen of your mind. Repeat the words of loving kindness to them three times.

Lastly, bring to mind all beings everywhere, people you know, people you don't know, and people far and near. Say the words of loving kindness to all beings everywhere.

When you are ready, open your eyes and continue with your work.

There are two parts to Step Eight: the creation of your list and the willingness to make amends. You have just completed the preparation for your list making. The practical part of this step is to glean the names of people from your previous work.

Refresh yourself by looking at the work you did on the previous steps and list any names here.

Did you include your own name on this list? If not, please add it now.

There may be some hiccup, or impedance, as you go to place a name on your list. You may have some residual reservation, rationalization, or resentment. If that is the case, make a star or other mark near the name and remember to work on those.

The obstacles of ego, false understanding, aversion, and even attachment may be at work here. Are there any names from your Fourth Step you have decided not to include here? Is there a name you have written down but he or she still holds hurt and harm in your heart, and you think you will never be able to apologize for your actions with him or her?

Describe how your ego (your outer sense of self) could stand in your way? What work are you willing to do to break through your ego?

Is there some misunderstanding or illusion about a situation that would prevent you from including someone? How would you amend that? What steps can you take to "understand rather than be understood"?

Do you flat out want to avoid seeing or meeting with someone? Do you want to avoid bringing up a situation that feels too uncomfortable? What feelings come up for you when you think of these situations?

Are you more comfortable with difficult feelings than with friendly, perhaps vulnerable, feelings? Why or why not? Does the anger or resentment with that person feel safer than talking about your side of the issue(s)? Why or why not?

Thinking about the yamas and niyamas, do any of these come into play when making your list?

- Yamas: non-harming, non-lying, non-stealing, non-excess, non-attachment

- Niyamas: cleanliness, contentment, self-study, discipline, surrender

When it comes time to be willing to speak your truth, the throat chakra is of great importance. The throat chakra provides us with the strength to speak and hear the truth. It is the union of our mundane, or worldly, chakras, and the more ethereal ones—the third eye and the crown. This union is important as you are connecting with your body and emotions and working toward being closer to your true and spiritual self. Your willingness will come from your sense of connection and stability: experiencing your emotions in their right size, having a sense of composure and command, and accessing your compassion and forgiveness. These are qualities provided by your first four chakras: root, sacral, solar plexus, and heart. Check in to see if you have a good base to support you.

How do you prepare your throat chakra for speaking your truth? Singing and chanting are two wonderful ways to do this. *Kirtan* is a special call and response form of ancient music that can invigorate and tune your throat chakra. Chanting *om* over and over until the sound blends into a background of breath and physical sensations of sound and breathing works, too. A mantra, a phrase or word found by you or provided to you, repeated over and over can balance your throat chakra

and become a source for meditation. The following is a traditional chant, "Om Namah Shivaya," which has no exact translation, but an explanation of it appears in the book *Yoga Sutras of Patanjali* by Gary Kissiah.

> Om is a sacred sound that reflects the divine consciousness. Namah means adoration, respect, and devotion. Shiva is the name of the God Shiva. Namah Shivaya has five syllables, which represent the five sheaths (or koshas) that cover the true Self. These are the gross body, the pranic body, the mental body, the intellectual body, and the blissful body. The mantra reflects the journey of consciousness as it moves from the gross body to the blissful body and ultimately to God.

You can find long versions of an "Om Namah Shivaya" kirtan, or song, online, if you like or you can just chant the three words over and over. There is no wrong way and there is no wrong inflection or pronunciation if your intention is clear. With a list written from a clear heart, with no reservations and a willingness to go to any length, the Eighth Step will securely prepare you for the process of Step Nine.

POSE

If you choose to do the Supported Fish pose, you can refer to the process in Chapter Eight of *Yogic Tools for Recovery* or follow the guidance provided in a short video at www.centralrecoverypress.com.

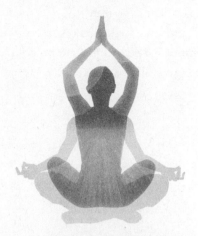

STEP NINE

We made direct amends to such people wherever possible,
except when to do so would injure them or others.

RECOVERY CONCEPTS

Justice, Responsibility, Acceptance of Consequences

GUIDING YOGIC PRINCIPLE

"When the yogi is firmly established in non-violence,
hostility is abandoned in his presence."

SUTRA 2.35

Sutra 2.35 is a powerful reference when applied to Step Nine. Amends are a path of non-violence, and their purpose is to make things right with others and within ourselves. Step Nine helps you get rid of the secrets, the pockets of pain that can erode your comfort in recovery. However, you don't sacrifice another's peace to serve your own, which takes discernment. Also, don't shirk what needs to be done with a false concern about harm; you have to be courageous and do the uncomfortable when it is right to do so. Advice and discussion are the sure way to ferret out the differences between the two extremes.

The ancients looked at the yamas, in fact all the qualities and actions, as occurring in the many levels of our being: thought, word, and action. When you look at your list of names from Step Eight, you may discover that some harms, or wrongs, were at the level of a thought, and others were in speech or deed, an action. There are occasions when there may have been a mixture of two or all three. That awareness may inform what type of amends you make.

Look at your list to see which type of amend or apology you will need to make. Don't think that you have to make these decisions alone. Connect with your sponsor or mentor. Take time as you consider each name. Decide which names require a direct apology, a letter or call, or need future actions and relations to be the amends. As you confer with your sponsor or mentor, begin to make a plan. Step Nine is a step of action.

As you consider the type of amend to be made, you may realize that there may be some people you cannot reach. They may have moved, or you may have never known their full names. Also, there may be people who have passed away.

You may have harmed or cheated a company, business, school, or some other organization. Amends may be difficult in these situations. Don't worry. There will be a process to address them all. Your sponsor can help you figure this out.

In this yogic process of investigating the steps, we go deep. Using the practices you learned while working the prior steps, contemplate how you feel at all levels of your being: body, mind, and spirit. Use the art of contemplation to investigate how you feel about the amends, how you propose to make it, and discern if you have any expectations about the results.

Look at your list. Take each name one at a time as you gain practice with the process. Start with the one that seems least challenging. Then repeat these sections for each person or institution.

Write down the name(s).

Recall specifically what you are making amends for.

Refer to your fourth-step inventory as well as your eighth-step list. Use the koshas to help guide you through the process of making amends.

When thinking about this person and the circumstances, how do you feel on a physical level? Do you have sensations in the pit of your gut? Any tightening of the shoulders or jaw? Any other physical sensation? Pause and note these sensations.

How do you feel on an energetic level? What is your breathing like right now?

Are you connected with your emotions? Are your emotions free or stuck? Do you experience feelings easily and smoothly, or do you have hiccups, numbness, or anxiety? Is there some other impedance to being in the present with the memories? Check in again with your physical layer and how it feels in your body as you remember this. Is there tightness anywhere?

What is the status of your intellectual layer, specifically the wisdom and discerning parts of you? Do you fall back to defenses or rationalizations? This is normal; just look at them and then move through them. Do you judge yourself harshly? Is there harming of self involved? Pause and see what you can do to let that go. The observing mind does not need to judge.

What is your spiritual connection? Evaluate your connection right now and going forward? Can you gain support and assistance from your higher power?

If you are finding difficulty in moving forward or falling into excuses, defenses, rationalizations, or any other form of denial or illusion, take some time to figure out where that is coming from. These resistances are rich in information and can help you understand yourself better. Rather than recoil or deny, look at them as an opportunity. You may not encounter resistance with the first name on your list but perhaps the second. Possibly, it will be your own name that conjures up some rationalization about why this cannot be done. Pause and hold yourself in compassion as you use the kleshas to investigate these forms of reticence. Overall consider if you have lingering misperceptions of the issues or incidences before you begin.

Do you know what the issue is and to whom the amends is due?

Is your ego involved in your hesitation? If so, explain how this shows up for you.

Are you craving a static, unaffected relationship or do you want the past to remain unchanged? Let sleeping dogs lie may be an attitude or approach you might have. Explain if you are experiencing this.

Do you want to avoid potential unpleasantness or discomfort, or do you want to evade or avoid a possibly disagreeable situation? Explain.

Is there fear? Are you concerned about the change in someone's perception of you? Are you concerned about his or her feelings if you bring attention to the issue(s)? Can you specify where the feeling of fear is coming from?

Are those fears having an impact on how, and if, you make the amends? If yes, explain how this shows up for you.

In the process of making amends, you are moving toward a more sattvic life, a life that is more harmonious inside as well as outside. The past can draw you down into the ignorance and delusion of tamas, but moving through rajas—not remaining in that movable or turbulent state—into sattva is the purpose of the steps. Step Nine is key to leaving the unconsciously or subconsciously harmful past behind you.

Avoiding harm of self and others is strongly recommended both in the words of the Ninth Step and in the practice of yoga. Before embarking on direct apologies in any form—phone, text, email, letter, or in person—look inward and be certain there will be no harm in the amends making, even considering if there will be harm in *not* making the amends. Take some time working it out with your sponsor or mentor. If you have questions, talk through the ramifications of direct amends. If direct amends are not possible, think of ways that reparations might be made in an indirect way. In this manner, you can continue to practice cleanliness—keeping your side of the street clean, as we say in recovery—doing what is yours to do and letting go of the result.

Allow yourself time between each amends making. Avoid skipping the previously outlined process. Not all questions will apply, but consideration of each will give you the opportunity to glean as much as possible from the process while it is fresh, while you are open.

This entire Ninth Step takes consistent energy and an internal focus on living a life in recovery. Help yourself employ the yogic practice of concentration and contemplation by learning Sutra 1.32: "The practice of concentrating on a single principle counteracts the obstacles." The following commentary by Reverend Jaganath Carrera provides you with guidance.

> We need that kind of one-pointed perseverance to overcome obstacles, and pierce the veneer of ignorance. We should never give up. Many people quit when they are on the brink of success. Determination always pays off. Ants, daily walking the same path across a stone wall, will wear a groove in it one day. Likewise, our practices will eventually eradicate ignorance.

Read and reread Sutra 1.32 and its commentary and apply them to the Ninth Step when you encounter an obstacle to completing the work. In this process, go into the mind for the reasons and into the body for the felt-sense objections. They both have something important to offer. Keep listening and working through the information. Take your time. This step is for you. Step Nine will help cleanse the wounds of the past and make the path forward much more rewarding and compassion filled.

POSE

Standing Mountain is a pose you should practice before each contact in your amends-making process. This can be a slow meditation to connect and integrate yourself as you find the resource of your inner dignity. If you choose to do the Standing Mountain pose, you can refer to the process in Chapter Nine of *Yogic Tools for Recovery* or follow the guidance provided in a short video at www.centralrecoverypress.com.

Stand up with arms released at your sides. Starting at the soles of your feet pull energy up through your feet drawing energy from the middle of the earth, imagining the fire and layers of minerals, rocks, and life coming up into your body. Engaging the muscles of the legs (be as specific as you can be as you draw your attention and energy through your limbs) and continue up to your torso. Front and back; engage your muscles lightly and firmly, back and front, right side, left side, breathing and aligning, integrating and finding union between posture and breath. Soften the shoulders, balance the head on the neck; eyes are level with the horizon, held in dignity.

Observe the area just above the crown of your head and imagine your source of energy, your higher power. Between earth and sky, you are balanced and grounded as you do Standing Mountain. You can proceed with your amends making with integrity.

After each amends has been made, find time to absorb the energy exchange resulting from that action or activity. Perhaps now is the time to go to a restorative yoga class to be guided and soothed, so you can let go completely, allowing your body to recover from the experience.

Do the practices of Standing Mountain and self-care each and every time you make an amends to ground yourself and honor your efforts as you do the Ninth Step. These will then be known activities to you, available when you need to call on them as you do your Tenth Step.

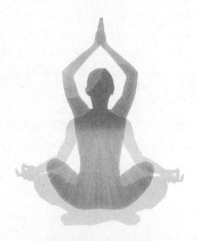

STEP TEN

We continued to take personal inventory
and when we were wrong promptly admitted it.

RECOVERY CONCEPTS

Perseverance, Maintaining Vigilance

GUIDING YOGIC PRINCIPLE

"By the dedicated practice of the limbs of Yoga,
the impurities are destroyed, the light of wisdom dawns,
and discriminative discernment is realized."

SUTRA 2.28

After the previous steps of hard work, you have arrived at Step Ten. Rather than looking back at your distant past of active addiction, you may find relief in being able to look at life in small doses: one day at a time. You are back to the present, and it is a lovely place to be. The excavation and examination of your life in relation to the issue set forth in Step One has been courageous. It has also been difficult and perhaps, at times, tedious. Now, practicing the niyama of cleanliness, you can keep up-to-date on those things you have done well and those that may need a do-over. Step Ten provides the format for this review.

Some people take the Tenth Step throughout the day; others make it a nightly practice to assess the day, or they take a personal inventory every so often when they think they might need a tune-up. Using the niyama of discipline, a sponsor could recommend early in your recovery that a regularly scheduled Tenth Step might be in order.

The observances of cleanliness, self-study, and discipline are guides in the practice of a regular Tenth Step. Consider if they are applicable for you.

Reflect on the values of keeping your side of the street clean, keeping your relationships straightforward and honest, and being clear in your communications as you do Step Ten. How did you do today?

Self-study includes using outside writings and wisdom. Do you have any books of quotations or resources that you use on a daily basis to keep your spirits up and your values intact? What are they?

Do you set aside a special time to do Step Ten? If so, when is it?

What is your challenge to making this a regular practice, if you find it difficult?

The yamas are a fantastic tool to evaluating your day. They cover many of the areas that can be troublesome. In thought, word, and action, how were you in relation to these five goals? Include both positive and negative.

- Non-harming (can include everything from words said in anger or gossip to negative thoughts and self-criticism)

- Non-lying (exaggeration, minimizing, false statements)

- Non-stealing (time, attention, stealing the limelight or words from someone's mouth)

YOGIC TOOLS FOR RECOVERY WORKBOOK

- Non-excess (greed)

- Non-attachment (letting go)

The kleshas are also rich ground for a quick check of your daily inventory. These may be more subtle, such as an underground stream that propelled an overreaction or harsh words to pop out. You may have felt these obstacles and avoided acting in an unwise way. You may have experienced one of them, acted or spoken to others without thought, and regretted the interchange. On later reflection, you might have discovered what was going on inside you. Sometimes we reenact and sometimes we avoid action, but often there is something else going on. The kleshas could be the source of that something else.

Did you suffer from false understanding or ignorance? Give examples.

Were you aware of your false ego or erroneous sense of self? What action or event made you aware of this?

Did you have a craving for or attachment to some particular response or outcome? What was it?

Did you want to avoid anything, such as a conversation, a job, or an outcome? What were your reasons for this?

Did you have a fear of something changing or ending? How does this show up for you?

You may have faced any of these obstacles over the course of the day. You may have approached them with wisdom and responded in alignment with your recovered self. Or, you may have acted in a way you wish you had not. In the latter case, amends making will need to be determined in support of promptly admitting it. You don't have to declare why you are doing this, merely what was wrong.

You may have your own name on your amends list from Step Eight. The Tenth Step is one way to approach this amends on a daily basis. Using the chakras and your koshas as guides to check in with yourself is a quick way to look at all your energy centers and needs without forgetting any area. Doing this on a regular basis may help you deepen your relationship with yourself—your true self—as you gain time in recovery.

How did you do today acknowledging your physical sensations, reactions, and needs? Did you eat when hungry? Did you take a pause in the day from time to time? Did you stay hydrated? Did you do some form of exercise?

How did you address your energetic needs? Were you aware of your breathing, or lack of breathing, at any point during the day? If you were aware of fatigue, did you rest? Were you able to go outside at any point in the day and get *prana*, or life energy, from the source, the sun?

How was your emotional body, the mental body that records impressions from your life? Were you triggered in the day? Describe those triggers and how you responded to them.

Did you react to something because of a historical recollection rather than the event of the moment? Were your feelings tender and sensitive, or did you feel robust and right sized?

Were you drawn into judgment or were you discerning today? Was your ability to watch and observe intact, or did comparison or preference cloud your view of things?

Did you take time today to connect with your universal spirit or higher power? Was there time today to check in with your spiritual self? How did you achieve these actions?

Pause here in your process and breathe. There's a lot to consider, and it may seem overwhelming. Know that you may not do it all every day. You may choose a tool or two each day to review your inventory. Know that with practice the series of questions become a little more automatic and a little easier to ponder. As challenging moments come up during the day, you may reach for some of these concepts and take a moment to choose how you will respond in light of what you have practiced. If you have a confrontation with a coworker, you may be able to pause and consider why it is bothersome and how you will respond, if at all. You can do a quick internal check, breathe, and choose.

MEDITATION

Before moving on to the chakras as a check-in tool, try a quick meditation. It can refamiliarize you with the chakras and remind you about some of the gifts a balanced chakra can provide. Read the following text all the way through once before you begin, remembering what you can, or have a friend read it to you while you take the journey from the root to the crown chakra.

Set an intention for the next few minutes to embody an awareness of your chakras. This is a way to become familiar with their sense and meaning. Begin with getting situated and comfortable. Let go of the world around you and be comfortable in your seat. You can center your gaze on a distant object or you may close your eyes.

Prepare yourself as you would for any meditation, paying attention to your seated position, your posture, and your breath. Take a few moments here to affirm your intention to bring your attention inside and feel your way through this process. Let go of outside inputs.

—Pause—

Take a moment to be sure that you are physically comfortable: no hairs tickling the cheek, no clothes pulling at you. Place your hands in your lap. Breathe in and out. Again.

In this brief journey through the chakras, repeat bringing the beam of your awareness to the swirling energy that is centered at each chakra. We will go through them highlighting what some of their gifts are. Know that there is no right way or wrong way to feel or to interpret your chakras. This is a journey to see what is, with curiosity and without judgment.

Bring your attention to your root chakra. Located at the base of the spine; this sphere of energy goes down the legs to the soles of your feet and rises up to the base of your spine. This is the energy of survival; it helps you determine if you are lonely, hungry, or tired. It is also the space of your connection to resources and support. This is your most elemental nature that guides you through the discipline of the mundane aspects of daily life.

—Pause and consider your connection here—

Moving to the sacral chakra located at the sacrum, which is in line with your hipbones. This is an area of intimacy and emotions as well as creativity and motion. This is a source of pleasure and pain—what you move toward and what you move away from. When in balance, you can look inside without fear and process emotions without judgment. How do you experience your sacral chakra today?

—Pause—

The solar plexus chakra gives you a sense of your personal power. Located just above the navel, the belly, this is the space in which you connect with your skills and abilities. It is also where you find your self-esteem and self-worth. You can gain energy to put your creativity into action when the solar plexus chakra is in balance. This can be the location of your gut brain and deeper instinct as well. Do you feel connected with your skills and abilities with adequate self-esteem? Breathe and check in.

—Pause—

Bring your attention to the heart energy center. This chakra is a source of love, compassion, and forgiveness, which provides us with our ability to transcend our ego. It is also where we acknowledge opposites, dark and light, male and female, inner and outer consciousness. The heart chakra also impacts our breath. Take a few breaths now to connect with your heart chakra.

—Pause—

The throat chakra is the conjunction of your earthly chakras and your spiritual ones. We hear and speak truth from this energy space. Listening acutely to what is being shared with you is a gift of the throat chakra. This is also where you begin to express your creativity. Take a moment now and check in with your throat chakra today.

—Pause—

Located above and between your eyes is the third eye chakra. Your ability to look inward and look outward, to discern patterns you find in life—behavior, emotions, and so on—is generated by the third eye chakra. It provides you with your intuition and helps order your thoughts. Take a few breaths now to check in with your third eye chakra.

—Pause—

Cupping the top of your head and reaching skyward with a thousand petals is the crown chakra. Thought and consciousness are governed by the energy in the crown chakra. This is where you witness your insides and the world around us. It is a lamplight to your spiritual being. How connected are you to this energy now?

—Pause—

Bring your attention now to the room around you and to your body. Become rooted once again to your seat. With intention, open your eyes and begin.

Use the following series of questions as a quick check in with your chakras. Think of it as an internal review of how you are doing now and if you have any leftover information from your day that you have not yet addressed.

What did you discover about your root chakra? How grounded and connected do you feel?

What about your sacral chakra? What awareness did you have?

Did you discover anything when bringing your awareness to your solar plexus chakra?

How is your heart chakra today?

Were you able to get in touch with the balance of your throat chakra?

Consider your third eye chakra. What awareness did you find there?

How is your connection with your crown chakra today?

As you make a practice of your Tenth Step, you can decide when to do it—daily, each evening, on the spot, or on an ad hoc basis—and you can practice it deeply doing all the series of questions described previously or select one or two paradigms to delve into your day. Remember to include what worked well in addition to discovering if there are any apologies or acknowledgements that need to be made to others. This is a very useful step and can help prevent relapse when taken seriously with full intentions.

POSE

If you choose to do the Swinging the Torso from Side to Side pose, you can refer
to the process in Chapter Ten of *Yogic Tools for Recovery* or follow the guidance
provided in a short video at www.centralrecoverypress.com.

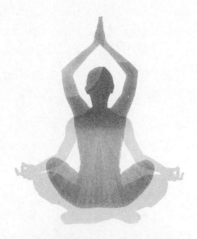

STEP ELEVEN

We sought through prayer and meditation to improve our
conscious contact with God *as we understood Him*,
praying only for knowledge of His will for us
and the power to carry that out.

RECOVERY CONCEPTS

Spirituality, Reflection

GUIDING YOGIC PRINCIPLE

"Liberation is attained when the mind becomes
as pure and as tranquil as the inner self."

SUTRA 3.36

Prayer and meditation with moments of quiet calm taken as a regular, disciplined practice can anchor your day and become a ballast for your life. One of the gifts of the steps, one of the many, is self-care. The first three steps lay a foundation for leaving the madness behind and gaining a partner, a higher power, in your journey to waking up to your inner true self. The next six steps help weed the garden of your being so that the goodness has room to grow. You begin to tend that garden on a regular basis in Step Ten. And now, in Step Eleven, you can bring in the beauty of nature to help it grow, allowing in the sunlight of the spirit.

You are the conduit; you send out prayer and bring in meditation. In the Eleventh Step, you learn to refine those skills so that you can be astute as you listen and clearer as you ask. It is self-care that grounds your new life in recovery.

Recovery from anything is hard, and the more discerning you become in your life purpose the more refined your connection with your higher power becomes. While this step concerns the practice of meditation, it is also about the practice of concentration, inward and outward connection, and a trust of intuition and inner knowing.

There is no official way to send out prayers, no perfect way to meditate. Many types and styles were presented in Chapter Eleven of *Yogic Tools for Recovery* and a few of them are listed here.

Prayer has many forms: a specific plea for self, a petition for others, a poem or refrain sent out to your higher power to give you guidance. One style or process may work one day, and you may choose an alternate on another day.

Meditation also has several doorways through which to enter that state. You can listen to external guides in the form of organized group meditation and online resources for guided meditation or you can focus on sounds. The breath is a common anchor to focus and refocus your wandering mind and attention. Using a phrase or word, silently repeated to yourself, can also keep your attention inward and your focus away from becoming involved in mental wanderings. Scanning the sensations in your body can also keep the mind from perseverating on any certain topic and allow it to remain in the present moment. Counting thoughts, using visualizations, or a practice such as a specific loving kindness, or metta practice, can all be in your toolbox. Trying these tools and being willing to change from one to another if you find difficulty with your usual practice can help you stay on the path.

Surrender is a big part of this step. Having an expectation that there will be any regular or specific outcome is perilous because you might think of things in terms of right and wrong, successful or unsuccessful. These are only concepts that will deter you from a regular practice.

STEP ELEVEN

Do you have expectations about what prayer should be like? Describe.

Do you have an assumption about meditation? If so, what is it?

Initially, you may need some assurance in order to be sure the type of meditation you are using is correct, perhaps signs in the form of found notes, sparking rocks, or overt events in the world that indicate you are on the right path. We don't get those. While many of us do get "God-shots" or "mini miracles"—those chance incidents or events during the day that wake us up—they may not be specific to the question or concern we have in mind. With regular practice you can also find a little more ease in your day, a little less criticism of self and others, and a little more ability to pause and reflect. These are the subtle signs of a regular meditation practice.

What kind of signs have you found as the result of your *current* practice of prayer and meditation?

Let yourself be open. Do not ask for anything in particular during prayer and avoid listening for something specific in meditation. The messages may be specific but more often they are broader, cultivating you for the day to come.

How can you approach Step Eleven? Some people start with inspirational readings. Do you have any books that you read for encouragement and motivation? What are they?

Using the niyama of discipline, can you commit to a certain time of day to practice your Eleventh Step? When would that be?

Can you attend to this on a regular basis? A particular length of time such as a week? What commitment can you make?

You are an integrated whole—body, mind, and spirit—and in this step you focus your energies on the spiritual. This is the innermost layer of the koshas, translated often as the bliss layer. Imagine being able to allow your bliss layer to be unencumbered by "shoulds," free of the burden of expectations. Let your bliss layer just be, so it can roam and bring you messages from your higher power.

Can you imagine doing that? What would impede you?

As you venture into the world of prayer and meditation, you will engage the energies of your sixth and seventh chakras: the third eye and the crown. When you have difficulty praying, when you have difficulty meditating—and you will, we all do—you can do practices to soothe and balance these two chakras. If you have trouble bringing your intuition and your connection to the cushion or chair or wherever or however you are praying and meditating, check out your other chakras. Perhaps you are not grounded, your emotions are flying around, or you are feeling off kilter, out of control, or a lack of mastery in your life.

Check in with your heart and throat chakras. Do you have some stone in your heart, something that is weighing you down? How does that show up for you?

Do you feel unheard, or have you not been listening to others? What actions can you take to be more present?

Use the practices set out in the preceding chapters to align yourself. They don't have to be too arduous and they don't have to take too long. Take a brief cruise inside yourself to see what might be standing in your way of taking a few moments to listen to your higher power and settle the fluctuations of your mind.

The second part of Step Eleven asks you to align yourself with what you need to do in this day to support your higher purpose and have the way cleared for you to do that. That is indeed a tall order. How are you supposed to know that? Consulting with your ethics, values, and your desire to be of service, the path will be laid before you. Do your footwork and let go of the rest. If you find yourself forcing your will, a circumstance or a person, into your own idea of how things should go, check in with your higher power. Is this in alignment with your higher power's will for you? Are you overreaching for the "power to carry that out"? When stuck or in emotional difficulty, you may find that it is a sign and a pause for reflection might be in order.

After having worked the previous steps, you may be more accurate about your intuition, separating it from impulse. You may be more secure in how you perceive things and feel more confident in your skills in the world. You may, however, find a little difficulty as you add prayer and meditation. Here are some practices to help you sit and listen.

Sometimes it is beneficial to do your personal yoga practice first before sitting down to read, ponder, ask, and listen. A personal yoga practice doesn't have to last for an hour, and it doesn't have to be rigorous or challenging, although it can be all of those. Often a mindful series of stretches, with attention to the breath and to the sensations in the body, can be your practice. Moving the spine forward and back, side to side, and in gentle twists is a great start. This can be enhanced by gentle movements in all the joints and concluded with a few minutes of savasana. You can even do these from a seated position. Take a few moments and try that now. Without a script or specified sequence, just move your body. After that, perhaps, sitting in prayer and meditation will be possible.

> Take a moment now to see if some prayer, some "ask," occurs to you. Perhaps a prayer for the health of another, relief for the difficulty that a sponsee is facing, or something that you need help and support with. This is your prayer. Include it here.

Now, select a type of meditation. Perhaps, you will go online to find some music, nature sounds, or a guided meditation, or you will be ready to sit in silence and use the counting of your thoughts or the rhythm of your breath.

What type of meditation are you going to use?

How much time can you commit to this period of prayer and meditation. There is no magic number, no minimum, no maximum, just a commitment. What will that be?

Set a timer so you won't have to keep checking. Give yourself into the practice, including your intention for prayer and your style of meditation. You will write about your experience afterward. Begin now.

What was your experience? Take a few moment to delve into the koshas.

- Physical layer: Was it hard to be still? Were you uncomfortable? Were you able to let go and settle in?

- Energy layer: Was your breath even? Did it provide you with an anchor? Were you conscious of your breath?

- Mental/Emotional layer: Were you aware of your feelings? Did you feel resistance, frustration, calm, or peace? Something else?

- Wisdom layer: Did you get any backtalk or other commentary? Did you experience the impartial observer of your inner self? Were you aware of the witness mind in any way?

- Bliss layer: Were you able to connect with your higher power? Was there any sense that your awareness was coming from some place other than your mind? Could you feel connection, a sense of being able to turn over your concerns?

The Eleventh Step is truly a step of practice. No two experiences are the same, although you may have similar experiences from time to time. Practice the setting of the intention as you did previously with your prayer and committing yourself, for today, to a certain type of meditation. Then sit for a specific amount of time. Tomorrow, practice again.

In addition to the still practices described previously, anything you do mindfully—hike, walk, cook, wash, and so on—can be done with concentrating on that process only thus becoming a meditation. You can do prayer and meditation together or separately. It is the discipline of intention setting and mindfulness that sets the practice apart from other things you do.

Once you get your ideas and the process comfortably in your body and mind, you may notice that you are able to practice meditation anywhere at any time. If you are unable to meet your prescribed moments in the morning, you can take a short time in your vehicle before going into your work or focus for a few moments at your desk or at lunch. Pause at anytime during your day to set an intention, focus on something, such as the horizon, the sky, or your breath, and let yourself be for two minutes. It takes about two minutes to settle in and let go. Open the doors of your mind and let the calming breeze of your universal connection with all beings flow and know you are not alone.

POSE

If you choose to do the Seated Position pose for your meditation, you can refer to the process in Chapter Eleven of *Yogic Tools for Recovery* or follow the guidance provided in a short video at www.centralrecoverypress.com.

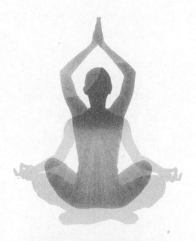

STEP TWELVE

Having had a spiritual awakening as the result of these steps,
we tried to carry this message to addicts,
and to practice these principles in all our affairs.

RECOVERY CONCEPTS

Service, Helping Others

GUIDING YOGIC PRINCIPLE

"On the destruction of impurity by the sustained practice
of the limbs of Union, the light of knowledge
reveals the faculty of discernment."

SUTRA 2.28

You are now on the path of awakening. It may come in glimpses, or you may have a sustained period of being in touch with the divine. It is from these moments of inspiration that you bring the best of yourself into service with others. You move out of the meetings and off the yoga mat to meet life on life's terms and to be of use to your fellows.

Are you ready to take your awakening into the world?

Listening to people share at meetings and, perhaps, reflecting on your own experience, you may have discovered that waking up is not a one time thing. There is more than one type of spiritual experience. Now, some seventy-three years after the first of the twelve-step programs was launched, we understand a little more about the variety.

What was or is your spiritual awakening like?

Do you have mini-awakenings, or mini-miracles, that refresh your connection to your spiritual guide? Describe how these show up in your life.

Can you recall one big "wake up"? An event that showed you were on the right path, or a moment that allowed you to recognize that you are part of a universal whole?

Are you worried that you won't experience a spiritual awakening? Or that somehow you are lacking or have been doing something wrong?

Don't be worried if you haven't had a big "aha" moment; you are here now and have been working toward a closer relationship with yourself and others. A huge step forward is walking in companionship with your spiritual guide.

Yoga is a way to find a visceral connection to one's spiritual self. It is also a way to begin to control the mind. Control of the breath can bring control of the mind, and control of the mind can bring about a way to continually realign yourself with the ethics, values, morals, and wisdom of your deeper, truer seed self—your atman.

Take a few moments here to recall the steps you have completed. Perhaps, take a moment to read through all the preceding eleven steps. Recall the yamas and the niyamas. Reacquaint yourself with the koshas, the kleshas, and the chakras. Think about the qualities of tamas, rajas and sattva. Now, turn your awareness inside. When you consider the benefits of the steps, where can you *feel* these principles?

> Using the breath as your centering guide, begin with the yamas and the niyamas. Can you bring sensory awareness to the ideals of non-harming, non-lying, non-stealing, non-excess, and non-attachment? Can you feel this in your body? If so, where? This can be a tug, a sense of neutrality, or even a release and peaceful sensation. How can you, or do you, take these into your daily life?

Where can you feel the observances of cleanliness, contentment, self-study, discipline, and surrender? Each may reside in a different place. What benefits do these provide you when you work with others?

Each step can bring a different feeling. Perhaps each step touches you in a different way. The experience can be felt over the entire body, or it can be localized. It is what it is with no expectation. Again, think about the result of these steps now considering your koshas.

How can being in touch with your koshas support you in your family and job or when you are in service?

How can being in touch with your energy layer help you in these areas?

How are you feeling in your emotional/mental layer? Is there an emotional flavor at your job right now? Are you wondering and considering? Worrying or impatient? How can checking in with this layer help you off the mat and out of the meetings rooms of recovery?

Your judgment mind may be super active right now: "Do I have a feeling? Is it the right feeling? What if I don't have a feeling? Is that wrong?" Or you could be evaluating: "I wonder if other people have written down more? Am I not getting it?" You are. Don't worry. You are exactly right where you need to be when you take the time to check in. That is the secret—checking in.

What is your wisdom layer telling you now?

Have you experienced some enlightenment in regards to the sufferings and obstacles—the kleshas? Have you had some experience pausing to discern the false from the real? In what way may this be useful in your life?

Practice the skill of taking a moment to consider internal reactions and external responses. Internal emotions have an impact on our external responses. Take time to sense how you are feeling. When you experience attachment or aversion it could impact your relationships with others.

Which tools can you use to identify and address the impacts of the kleshas?

Has working the steps with these concepts helped you discover occasions of false ego? Do you have a process to check in with your ego on an ongoing basis? Can monitoring this obstacle help you in your work, with your family, and so on?

Has fear of change, or of transformation, been observed and addressed? Will this awareness help you as you work with others?

Has understanding the kleshas helped you apply the steps in daily life? How?

Finally, take a closer look at the chakras. See if you can write about the influence the chakras have had on your understanding of the steps or perhaps the other way around.

Describe how the steps have helped you understand how important balanced chakras are to a harmonious life.

Go through all seven chakras and see if evaluating the balance of each can or has helped you "practice these principles in all [your] affairs." Refer to the chart at the end of this workbook to refresh your memory.

- Root chakra

- Sacral chakra

- Solar plexus chakra

- Heart chakra

- Throat chakra

- Third eye chakra

- Crown chakra

How can you muster this huge compendium of insight and recovery that you have created about yourself, your experience, and your growth to assist you in your service to others? How can you keep this work alive and the discoveries available to you throughout your day?

In what ways does this work better prepare you to be *you* when you are in a position to sponsor or provide support to another person in, or looking for, recovery?

POSE

If you choose to do the Tranquility pose, you can refer to the process in Chapter Twelve of *Yogic Tools for Recovery* or follow the guidance provided in a short video at www.centralrecoverypress.com.

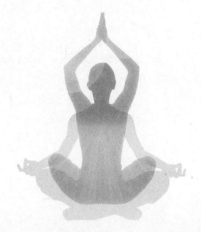

PUTTING IT ALL TOGETHER

You have worked the steps in a new and unique way and taken the time and effort to include a new paradigm while working the traditional steps. The universal principles of the steps allow for personal experience and application to any and all manifestations of addiction, as well as compulsions and obsessions. This special pair of yogic glasses is only one way to examine the steps. You have chosen it and completed the work. Take a moment to pause and breathe in the joy of this accomplishment.

What final words do you have to offer yourself now that you have completed this process?

Siddhartha by Hermann Hesse, is a story about Govinda and Siddhartha, which was the Buddha's name before he became the enlightened one. It has a powerful sentence in its early pages. The translation of that sentence went something like this: "The target of the arrow is the bow." I took that to mean that our heart, our soul, is the real thing on which the aim of our efforts should focus.

Look to strengthening and clarifying your heart and all goodness will follow you on your true path.

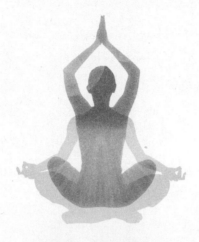

KEY TERMS

For a full explanation of these terms and deeper explanation of their meaning, please refer to the introduction of *Yogic Tools for Recovery: A Guide to Working the Twelve Steps*. These word and phrases are noted here to remind you about what the words refer to. The expanded explanation in the book along with the illustrations can help you as you use this workbook.

Bhastrika breath: bellows breath. A breath with a forceful exhale and then a forceful inhale through the nostrils—equal energy in both directions. Repeat ten or twenty times or for a full minute or other defined sequence.

Chakras: the energy wheels or discs within us

- **Root**: the center of grounding and support

- **Sacral**: the center of intimacy and creativity

- **Solar plexus**: the center of self-control, skills, and self-esteem

- **Heart**: the center of compassion, forgiveness, and connection

- **Throat**: the center of listening to and speaking our truth

- **Third eye**: the center of self-awareness and inner vision

- **Crown**: the center for imagination, realism, and spiritual connection

Gunas: energetic qualities in all things
- **Tamas**: the qualities of inertia, darkness, and heaviness

- **Rajas**: the qualities of movement, action, and change

- **Sattva**: the qualities of harmony, purity, and balance

Kleshas: the obstacles or sufferings
- **Avidya**: false understanding; seeing the unreal as real; the impermanent as permanent

- **Asmita**: ego; the misunderstanding of who we are

- **Raga**: attachment to pleasure; craving

- **Dvesha**: avoidance of pain, rejection, or discomfort

- **Abhinivesha**: fear of death or transformation; change

Koshas: the layers of our being
- **Anamaya**: the physical layer

- **Pranamaya**: the energy (breath) layer

- **Manomaya**: the emotional/mental layer

- **Vijnanamaya**: the wisdom layer (the observer)

- **Anandamaya**: the spiritual or bliss layer

Metta meditation: a specific style of meditation where you wish kindness, health, and healing to people close, near and far, yourself, and even those with whom you have difficulty. It is a practice of forgiveness and compassion.

Niyamas: the observances, or the internal practices, which are considered at all levels: thought, word, and deed

- **Saucha**: cleanliness/purification

- **Santosha**: contentment, acceptance, and gratitude

- **Tapas**: discipline and purification through self-control

- **Svadhyaya**: self-study and benefiting from life's lessons

- **Ishvara pranidhana**: turning it over, surrender to a higher power, selfless action

Pranayama: breathing practices designed to enhance life and vitality

Samskara: the grooves of habitual thinking; the automatic, historical and possibly conditioned response to life

Ujjayi breath: a regularly paced breath that is expelled through a slightly constricted throat. Both the inhale and the exhale are through the nose. There may be a slight audible sound sometimes referred to as Darth Vader in style.

Yamas: the restraints; the behaviors we resist and desist in life and in recovery

- **Ahimsa**: non-harming; self or others, in actions or in thought

- **Satya**: non-lying; to live and speak our truth one day at a time

- **Asteya**: non-stealing; avoid taking anything—property, reputation, consideration, or care—and do not take anything that is not freely given

- **Brahmacharya**: non-excess; to live modestly in all ways

- **Aparigraha**: non-attachment; avoid greediness and attachment, keeping only what you need

STEPS, PRINCIPLES, AND EXAMPLE TIE-INS WITH YOGA

STEP	CONCEPT / PRINCIPLE	EXAMPLE TIE-IN
1	*Honesty*: It is vital to concede that we are addicts if we are to achieve recovery. The odds are against us if we don't completely admit defeat and surrender. This takes being truthful with ourselves. The actively using addict cannot differentiate the true from the false. By learning to be honest with ourselves and admit an honest desire to be in recovery, we begin the spiritual program of action.	Ahimsa; ishvara pranidhana
2	*Hope*: In order to engage in a course of addiction recovery, we must have hope of success. If there is no hope, why try? We have not been able to stay clean, abstinent, or sober on our own, and the desperation we feel when we enter a twelve-step program can be overwhelming. A way to instill hope is to realize recovery is not a question of ability but rather a desire to stay abstinent. Seeing others recover and live free from addiction brings hope.	Freedom from samskara; possibility for change and health; sanity; saucha
3	*Faith*: This decision step to go on with the Twelve Steps asks that we step into faith. It is only a matter of being willing to believe. Through the process of the Twelve Steps, that belief turns into faith. We carry this faith into the rest of the steps by being willing to believe. We must begin to have faith it will work. We also believe that our universal spirit cares for us, that we are not alone.	Ishvara pranidhana; karma; avidya; asmita
4	*Courage*: This step is really about having the courage to honestly look at ourselves. Take a look at how our behavior has become warped to justify our continued addictive thinking and actions. We are here to take an honest assessment of ourselves. Looking at causes and conditions of our addictive or obsessive behavior can be scary. We are brave and can do this.	Kleshas; koshas; gunas; and chakras
5	*Integrity*: If we have truly done a thorough job of introspection and evaluation of our assets and shortcomings, do we have the integrity to own up to it? It can be difficult to be open and honest about our past behaviors. Sharing our past reminds us that we are not alone. In talking aloud about the past we begin to learn to do the right thing even though no one is watching.	Yamas; niyamas; finding guru; being student
6	*Willingness*: Now that we have accomplished an inventory of the good and not so good aspects of our character and behavior, are we willing to change them? All of them? The important part in this twelve-step principle is the willingness to let go of old behaviors and rely on our higher power.	Kleshas; investigate samskara

STEP	CONCEPT / PRINCIPLE	EXAMPLE TIE-IN
7	*Humility*: Here we move further into action. We have seen in Step Five where we have been selfish and self-centered. We practice being humble by realizing that we are not the center of the universe. We are all simply small parts of a huge whole. To be human is to make mistakes. Hopefully our journey has led us to the point where we can readily admit mistakes and accept ourselves for being imperfect. We are asking for help in forgiving ourselves.	Niyamas for rightsizing life and self, investigate asmita
8	*Brotherly Love*: While we prepare a list of those to whom we owe amends, it becomes time for the "golden rule." It is important to begin treating others as we wish to be treated. We must also learn not to judge others but accept them for who they are, not our vision of who they should be.	Chakra balancing
9	*Forgiveness*: We are continuing to remove the barriers that can block our progress in healing. We are actively sweeping our side of the street clean. We are learning to become accountable while making amends to those people we have harmed. We are practicing new behaviors by facing our wrongs, so it is important to have this self-discipline. We are trying to correct our wrongs through action, not just words. We stay close to our sponsor during each amends to stay focused, practicing compassion and forgiveness as we go.	Tapas; ahimsa; satya; aparigraha
10	*Perseverance*: We have entered the world of the Spirit and strive to grow in understanding and effectiveness. This takes practice and means we have to keep on keeping on. We are beginning to trudge the road of Happy Destiny, and this takes diligence.	Tapas; samskara; kleshas
11	*Spiritual Awareness*: Step Eleven suggests that we continue to improve our conscious contact with our higher power, so we tap into that power through prayer and meditation. We become cognizant of the blessings we are receiving in our new life. We learn to notice the handiwork of our higher power in all aspects of our lives.	Concentration; meditation; ishvara pranidhana; avidya; asmita
12	*Service*: Having experienced a psychic change that keeps us in recovery, one day at a time, we are empowered to demonstrate the new principles by which we live. We remain in action in our daily life through example. We seek out and are available to help others in need. We continue to carry the message of hope and recovery. We strive to help wherever we can even in the smallest, simplest tasks of life.	Seva; karma yoga; right action; teaching; witnessing (koshas) with sattva

HOW CHAKRAS AFFECT YOUR BODY

CHAKRA	OVERACTIVE	UNDERACTIVE	IN BALANCE	RIGHT / CHALLENGE
ROOT	Lethargic, overspending, feeling spacy, fearful, overeating, anxiety, overdependence on others	Undereating, restless, scattered thoughts, body image issues, procrastinating	Feeling supported, stability, trust, security, sense of connectedness to self and world	To be and to have / Fear
SACRAL	Emotionally explosive, taking risks, abusive self-destructive, difficulty letting go, obsessive thinking and behavior	Blocked creativity, difficulties with intimacy, risk averse, anxious, emotionally numb	Feel at home in body, able to connect with healthy pleasure, ability to tolerate the unknown	To feel / Guilt
SOLAR PLEXUS	Poor boundaries, overactive self-will and sense of personal power, misuse of power and control, prone to perfectionism	Fear of rejection, low self-esteem, fear of criticism, passive, sluggish	Peaceful, generous, healthy sense of personal power, self-respect, self-esteem	To act / Shame
HEART	Paranoid, poor boundaries, indecisive, overloving, overtrusting, denial of one's own needs	Withholding, self-pity, fear of loneliness, isolation, "heart scars"	Love, compassion for self and others, forgiveness, healthy relationships, connecting mind and spirit, joy, gratitude when "heart scars" are healed	To love and be loved / Grief
THROAT	Anger and sadness, rage, excessive talking, explosive utterances	Being timid, holding back, silence, fear of speaking, speech problems	Express thoughts and feelings clearly, source of positive energy and growth, honesty, truth, independence	To speak and be heard / Lies

CHAKRA	OVERACTIVE	UNDERACTIVE	IN BALANCE	RIGHT / CHALLENGE
THIRD EYE	Confusions, exaggerated imagination, day dreaming, living in fantasy, deluded thinking	Sensory difficulties, battle between intuition and intellect, poor memory, can't find patterns in actions and reactions	Clear vision, understanding inner self, trusting intuition, elimination of selfish attitudes, ability to discern the difference between truth and illusion	To see / Illusion
CROWN	Difficulty with sleep/wake cycle, depression, migraines, overly sensitive to sense stimulations, difficulty meditating, spiritual bypass, overly intellectual	Difficulty sleeping, isolation, difficulty learning, skepticism, alienation, hopelessness, disconnection from others and spirit	Inward flow of wisdom, enlightenment, dynamic thought, open to the divine, release of both over- and underactive mental reactions, live in the present moment, trust inner guidance	To know and to learn / Attachment

POSES TO ALIGN YOUR CHAKRAS

CHAKRA	YIN	YANG	HEALING HELP	AFFIRMATION
ROOT	Back lying pose with knees bent, or supported bridge with attention to the root chakra area	All standing poses with attention to the feet, all seated poses with attention to the seat	Walk barefoot, garden, walking or hiking, being with friends	I will be provided for. I have comfort and community.
SACRAL	Dragonfly forward fold, diamond butterfly forward fold	Squats, cobra pose	Baths, massages, yoga classes, artistic and crafts expressions	I have the right to have healthy boundaries. I am able to express myself creatively. I can experience the moment through my senses.
SOLAR PLEXUS	Deep supported twist, belly lying over a bolster	Lunge twist, revolved triangle	Cycling, hiking, taking photos, being a part of groups and taking leadership or service positions	I love and accept myself. I stand up for myself. I am worthy of love and respect.
HEART	Sphinx, seal, or melted heart pose, breathing bolster behind rib cage in "brook" pose	Hands clasped behind back forward fold, any of the standing heart opening poses	Spending time with loved ones or pets, dancing, partner yoga practices, child heart meditations	I forgive myself. I am grateful for the challenges that have helped me transform. I have the right to love and be loved.
THROAT	Supported fish pose, allowing the head to drop back	Fish pose, shoulder stand, head rotations, back bends	Chanting, singing, humming, listening to music and sounds	I am open and honest in my communications. I have a right to speak my truth. I know how to listen with compassion.

CHAKRA	YIN	YANG	HEALING HELP	AFFIRMATION
THIRD EYE	Supported child's pose, head on the ground or support	Balance poses, dolphin pose	Contemplation, visualization, Tai chi and other meditative movement practices	I am in touch with my inner guidance. I seek to learn from my past. I am open to inspiration and bliss.
CROWN	Savasana	Tree pose, savasana, head stand	Focus on joy, laughter, play, amusing movies, books, prayer, spiritual texts, connection to higher power	I honor the divine within me. I cherish my spirit. I love and accept myself as I am.

CHAKRAS AND THE TWELVE STEPS CORRELATION

CHAKRA	STEPS	REASONS
ROOT	1, 2, 3	Grounding, safety, "root to rise," moving on effectively begins with a strong base. Step One is to cease the activity; Step Two is to recognize return to health is possible; and Step Three is to be willing to connect with something (bigger) (other) than yourself. Lose fear and become willing to be and to have a life.
SACRAL	4, 6, 7, 10	You identify then ameliorate your chaos-oriented outlook, find appropriate intimacy, and work on a continual practice of self-evaluation for movement in a positive direction. Develop healthy feelings and let go of guilt.
SOLAR PLEXUS	2, 3, 4, 5, 10	Find health and healing and connection with your higher power and another person. You develop your skills in self-care, awareness, and growth. Acceptance and letting go can improve. Find "right action" and live without shame.
HEART	All	All steps lead toward forgiveness and compassion; focus on it here. By creating an open field of moving beyond duality, right/wrong, good/bad, you move toward a more loving experience of the world. You find your right to love and be loved, letting grief pass through you.
THROAT	4, 5, 8, 9, 10, 11, 12	As you learn to discover your truth through the steps, you share it with others and take action when needed. You also listen to hear the truth from others, the connection between your sensory input and your spiritual and intellectual input. You learn to speak and to listen and discern truth from lies.
THIRD EYE	4, 5, 6, 7, 11	You look inward and separate truth from fiction, the real from the unreal. You move from checking out your own actions according to your ethics and values and gain support from others as you change course to a better way of living. You maintain connection to your higher power to continue the process of growth and self-realization. You gain clarity in what you see and avoid illusions.
CROWN	10, 11, 12	Keep your side of the street clean, and do what is yours to do, letting go of the results and allowing joy and abundance in your life. As you practice learning and knowing, you also practice letting go. It is through letting go that you can find and embrace the new.